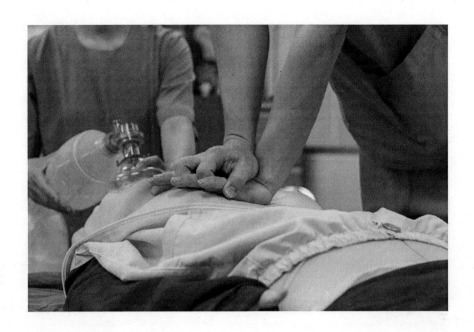

Becoming a Medical Educator

D1615255

**Professor Peter Donnelly &
Professor Derek Gallen**

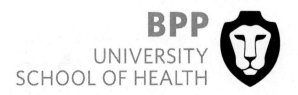

BPP
UNIVERSITY
SCHOOL OF HEALTH

First edition August 2017

ISBN 9781 5097 0763 8
eISBN 9781 5097 0767 6
eISBN 9781 5097 0771 3

British Library Cataloguing-in-Publication Data
A catalogue record for this book is available from
the British Library

Published by
BPP Learning Media Ltd
BPP House, Aldine Place
London W12 8AA

www.bpp.com/health

Printed in the United Kingdom

Your learning materials, published by BPP
Learning Media Ltd, are printed on paper
sourced from sustainable, managed forests.

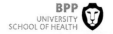

Contents

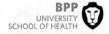

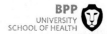

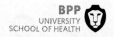

About the publisher

The UK's only university solely dedicated to business and the professions.

We are dedicated to preparing you for a professional career. We offer a strong commercial approach, within a business culture designed to help you stand out in the workplace after you graduate. Our programmes are designed in partnership with employers and respected professionals in the fields of law, business, finance and health.

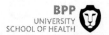

About the authors

Professor Peter Donnelly, MB BCH BAO FRCPsych BA(OU) FAcadMEd FHEA FRCPEdin MMed

Peter worked as a consultant psychiatrist in the NHS for 18 years with experience in all aspects of medical education from selection into medical school, undergraduate teaching delivery and curriculum development. He has also worked as an Associate Medical Director responsible for the ongoing CPD of all medical staff in an NHS Trust. He has worked in the Wales Deanery more latterly as Deputy Dean for 7 years and now as Interim Postgraduate Dean. In his Deanery roles he leads a range of medical education initiatives and is responsible for the quality management of training across all specialty curricula.

Professor Derek Gallen, BSc MB BS DCH DRCOG FRCGP FAcadMEd, FRCPEdin FHEA MMEd

Derek was a Postgraduate Dean who has a UK wide profile in the field of medical education. He has developed numerous educational initiatives and was the lead for the introduction of the Foundation Programme in the UK, academic placements, educational contracts and a founder member of the Academy of Medical Educators of which he went on to become president. He is currently the President of the Association for the Study of Medical Education (ASME).

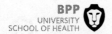

Acknowledgements

The authors would like to acknowledge the support of all colleagues, consultants, GPs, trainees and students who have helped to shape the narrative in this book. We thank the Academy of Medical Educators for use of their material and to BPP Learning Media for their support.

Peter would like to express his gratitude to family members for their support including Sheila and in particular, Paul and Stephen for their tolerance and good humour.

Derek would like to thank all the family, Paula, Luke, Alice, Tom and Isabella, Rachael, Johnny, Violet and Daisy for just being there.

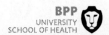

Foreword

If we're being honest about a career in medical education, many of us oldies have made it up as we went along, finding and taking opportunities for development as educators and leaders in a haphazard fashion. Donnelly and Gallen have written an authoritative book that provides a first class road map of the medical education career path for anyone, at any stage in their career, from medical studentship to dean of a medical school.

By tackling each aspect of the medical education and training career journey, they explore the options and the pathway through the complexities of medical structures, in a way that all can understand, using vivid illustrations of others' career experiences. Although this is an easily digestible and 'right good read', it is fleshed out with references to the key publications and theories that will allow the reader to explore the topics in more depth if they so wish. It can be dipped into for reference, yet also provides a clear overview of the opportunities available now and in the future.

This is an up to date snapshot of the world of medical education career paths and structures that should be read by all involved in the teaching and training of doctors, but especially to those with a hankering to navigate their way to a fulfilling career in developing both themselves and the generation of doctors coming behind. I hope others will enjoy it as much I did.

Professor W Reid MD FRCP (Glasg, Edin)
Dean of Postgraduate Medicine
SE Scotland and Chair COPMeD UK

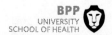

Chapter 1

Who is this book for?

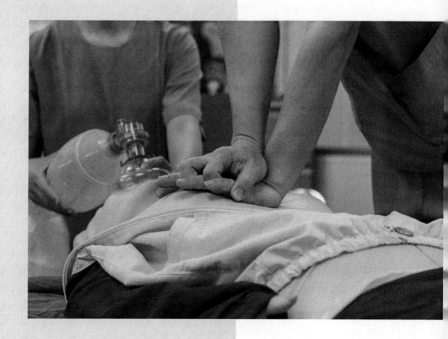

Chapter 1

Introduction

Although this book is entitled *Becoming a Medical Educator*, the principles and steps outlined will hopefully be relevant to a number of healthcare professionals.

The first thing to ask yourself is: why is a career in medical education attractive? It is important not only to realise the advantages as well as the challenges of moving into a career in medical education, but also to recognise how rewarding it can be to go from a portfolio career in education to a full-time role.

All doctors are trained over a number of years mapped to curricula, firstly undergraduate then postgraduate. The focus in general is on acquiring the skills, knowledge and competencies to deliver excellent clinical care to patients. All doctors, even early on in their career as medical students, will get involved in teaching peers and their juniors. As a doctor moves through their career pathway, opportunities arise for them to develop the skills commensurate with being a medical educator.

How to use this book

The chapters in this book focus on various aspects of the development and role of a medical educator. Some will be more relevant at certain points in your career. It is therefore important to dip into the various sections when they are most pertinent to your development.

All doctors will (and should) put clinical medicine first in terms of their career pathway, from qualifying at medical school and acquiring the Certificate of Completion of Training. However, a large part of the medical workforce are not in formal training programmes but still have a major role to play in teaching and training the National Health Service (NHS) workforce. This book is also highly relevant for them.

At any given point it is important to have a sense of a career plan. Revalidation is a significant driver for all doctors to focus on their current activity and consider appropriate continuing professional development (CPD). Doctors now have to revalidate against all of their roles. The more substantive a medical education role you move into, the greater the focus within the appraisal cycle on

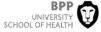

reflecting on those roles. This will also mean greater emphasis on CPD mapped to that educational role.

This book will help you to consider your current level of commitment to medical education and increase your understanding of the potential career pathways and opportunities that are out there. Hopefully, it will guide you with some practical steps, signposting qualifications, experience, knowledge and knowledge in action. All of the skills which are required when focusing on the medical education role are transferable; for example, leading teams, communication, curriculum delivery, research and sharing best practice. In this book we discuss the growing focus and demand by doctors for a portfolio career and how you can prepare and position yourself to move into those roles. These include a range of opportunities encompassing undergraduate, postgraduate, NHS, government and Royal Colleges.

Chapter summaries

Chapter 2: Career decision-making – portfolio careers

This chapter describes the growing interest in portfolio careers and highlights the advantages of such a career approach. It provides simple and practical tools you can use to help shape your career pathway. We also identify the risks of busy clinicians taking on a wide range of roles, which can lead to underperformance and therefore the need for you to consider funnelling down in your portfolios.

Chapter 3: Undergraduate medical education careers

This chapter aims to provide you with an overview of an education career in undergraduate medicine. We describe different levels of educational responsibility in a medical school and reflect on the national drivers that will shape your day to day activities such as the National Student Survey. We also focus on typical medical school activities that you may have responsibility for, such as curriculum design, assessment, admission policies and the importance of the links with the local NHS.

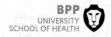

Chapter 1

Chapter 4: Postgraduate education careers

This chapter discusses the wide range of opportunities in the postgraduate medical education arena, including such roles as Education Supervisor, Training Programme Director and Head of Specialty School. We describe the links from postgraduate to medical schools and government.

Chapter 5: NHS, government and Royal College medical education roles

This chapter provides you with an overview of roles in the NHS from specialty based to Associate Medical Director for Education and the activities you will typically be involved in. We describe the links across all these areas into government and Royal Colleges.

Chapter 6: Prepare – which qualifications, why, when and where?

This chapter highlights the General Medical Council's (GMC) standards and the Academy of Medical Educator's domains that you can use to help steer your learning. There are in general two levels of learning: CPD and formal taught programmes such as a Master's in Medical Education and PhDs. There are other qualifications that can be useful in general such as a Master's in Business Administration. There are a range of providers that you can explore.

Chapter 7: Current frameworks in medical education

This chapter gives an overview of the GMC standards for undergraduate, postgraduate and NHS education and training. We cover key issues such as revalidation, the point of registration, less than full-time training and the generic professional capabilities.

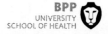

Chapter 8: Surviving as a medical educator

This chapter provides you with examples of individual and organisational tactics to use on a day to day basis to enhance your resilience. We describe organisational concepts that will help you manage and lead teams in a medical education arena such as decentralised decision-making. We identify support you can consider accessing, such as mentoring and executive coaching.

Chapter 9: The future of medical education in the workplace

This chapter gives you an overview of key issues in the future. We cover, amongst other issues, generalist training, the Medical Licensing Assessment and education contracts for trainees. Although this book is about becoming a medical educator, we stress the importance of a multiprofessional approach to education and training going forward.

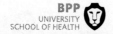

Chapter 1

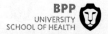

Chapter 2

Career decision-making – portfolio careers

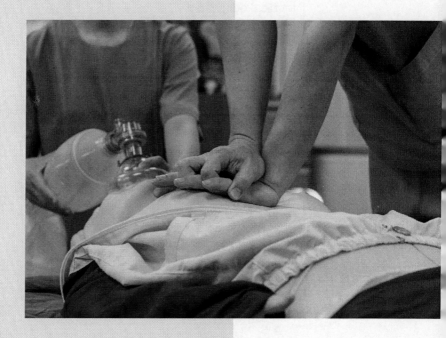

Introduction

A question to ask yourself is: what makes you tick? What do you enjoy? What do you get a buzz from? What is important to you?

Most doctors will get enormous satisfaction from clinical practice – that's what they trained for – but there is so much more that a degree in medicine qualifies you for and provides you with other opportunities.

Careers in medical education can be seen at different levels with different types of rewards and challenges and hence when deciding on which level it is useful to consider your drivers; what gives you positive feedback?

Clinical practice has never been the sole destination for medical training, with doctors diversifying into a range of roles inside and out of medicine; the arts, business and politics to mention a few. It is essential to realise that there are other avenues to explore but that it takes a positive step by you to seek out these opportunities. Box 2.1 provides a list of some potential portfolios for doctors.

Examples of portfolio careers

Research, lab based, clinical, social
Medical education
Management/leadership
Medico legal
Private clinical practice
Royal College
Journalism/media
Arts
Engineering
Technology
General Medical Council
Financial services
Aerospace
Aviation
Politics
Government
Health policy
Pharmaceuticals
Humanitarian/Medical volunteer work

Box 2.1 Examples of portfolio careers

Portfolio careers

Portfolio careers are not new in medicine and date back famously to the 19th century with Anton Chekhov who practised as a medical doctor throughout his career and started writing short stories as a means to increase his income.

So you ask; what is a portfolio career?

Charles Handy (1991) in his book *The Age of Unreason* describes the then emerging concept of the portfolio career. He sees a portfolio as a way of describing how different bits of your work all fit together. A portfolio enables you to have a more rounded approach to all aspects of your work. Handy describes five portfolio categories (see below) and suggests that if your income is sufficient to meet your needs that satisfaction can come from a portfolio of paid and/or unpaid work. This view chimes with Maslow's hierarchy of needs model which suggests that if your basic needs have been met, including financial security, then higher level needs can be sought after.

Portfolio roles can vary over time and work best if they meet the needs and wishes of the individual. Doctors whose portfolio career acts as a role model for those doctors in training and medical students have inspired a number of doctors to actively pursue the qualifications and experience required at a much earlier stage. Thus there is an increasing realisation of the benefits of a portfolio career and individuals are becoming proactive in the process of understanding their own changing career needs over their lifetime.

Handy's five categories

1. Wage (salary) work: money paid for time given

2. Fee work: money paid for results

3. Study work: taken seriously but is not recreation (eg learning a new language)

4. Gift work: work done for free outside of home

5. Homework: tasks you do at home, with the family and time outside of 1 to 4

Box 2.2 Handy's five categories

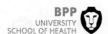

Most of us (but not all) enter medical school to become doctors with the ultimate aim of becoming a General Practitioner (GP) or Consultant, the 'autonomous clinician'. In the first few years after achieving that goal we typically focus our efforts on 'moulding the service', putting our own stamp on the clinical service for the direct benefit of patients. After we have achieved this, or as close to it as we can, there comes a point in your career that the clinical role alone may not be as challenging as it was at the beginning. This period of time is of course variable but is described in General Practice as a 'five years rule' and in secondary care as 'the seven-year itch' (Grey, 1996). At these points some of us will reflect and seek out more challenging roles. You develop and hone a considerable set of skills and talents as a clinician. A question for yourself is … will my 'core' clinical role be the best way for me to exploit/use those talents to the full over the lifespan of my working career?

Case study

I had been a principal in a busy city centre practice for four years. I was busy, very busy and the paperwork, the bureaucracy, was getting worse and worse. I thought about just dropping a few days, going part time, but honestly the cut in pay wasn't realistic. I thought of retraining in a specialty, to become a GP with a special interest. But the more I thought about it, that was just replacing one busy clinical role with another busy clinical role. I wanted to be busy, earn money and still contribute to medicine. I saw an advert for a new role in my local medical school, Assistant Director of Communication Skills. I decided to explore this and realised quickly that I had a lot of experience in this area and I was encouraged by my partners and family to apply.

The focus today, quite rightly, is the importance of a good work–life balance. This contrasts with the so-called baby boomers' career values. The baby boomer generation, born in the immediate post World War II period, 1946–1964, sees a well-defined linear career pathway with a career ladder and if you work hard you will progress up that ladder. Generally, baby boomers pursue a profession and stay in it for life, with job security and extrinsic rewards (eg financial). Their mantra is: 'I live to work.' Motivation is a complex construct but can be seen as what drives us to deliver … what drives us to act/behave in a certain way in regard to a

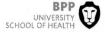

particular end/task. We can have high levels of motivation and different types of motivation.

Intrinsic	External
Do it for inherent satisfaction	Do for some external goal
Enjoyment	Money
Fun	Sanctions
Challenge	Regulated
Interesting to me	Fixed
Social worth	Social worth

Table 2.1 The differences between intrinsic and extrinsic motivation

Generation Y on the other hand, born between 1980 and 2000, see their career changing direction more frequently, bridging from one career path to another and having less security but more flexibility, and their focus is more on intrinsic rewards. This generation is also described as being more shaped by technology than the baby boomers. So the Generation Y career values include 'I work so I can live, I want to have fun.'

The traditional approach of a doctor qualifying as a GP or a Consultant and then continuing in that role for the rest of their working life, the linear career, is becoming less the norm. This applies to all professions and is driven by a number of factors. Portfolio careers can also suit employers as in general they prefer flexibility in their workforce and fixed-term contracts in medicine are now offered more often than was the case previously, as opposed to a 'job for life'.

So, combining clinical medicine with other roles is an increasingly important and frequent pathway. At its most basic level the portfolio career allows a blending or sequencing of roles, giving you job satisfaction, but must be tailored to meet your individual needs. Portfolio careers in medicine have been around in General Practice for many years but there is increasing interest from doctors in secondary care on this approach to careers. Why is this?

GP and Consultant roles have changed. As a doctor, respect has to be earned and is not a given right that may have been offered in previous generations as a result of the title. There is more litigation, reduced prestige, reduced public respect and the potential for reduced satisfaction with clinical practice.

The focus in medical school and on into postgraduate training is for you to acquire (to a greater extent) the clinical skills required to be able to perform as the autonomous clinician in your specialty. On the way to gaining those clinical skills Royal College exams and other hurdles such as workplace-based assessments have to be passed.

As a result, once the goal is achieved there is a risk of little forward planning for when that central clinical role doesn't provide the intellectual challenges it did previously. It could be argued that the current pressure on the need to deliver service in primary or secondary care places all doctors potentially in a position whereby the health organisations they are working in – Trusts, Health Boards or Practices – do not provide institutional support for doctors to develop other related interests in medical education, clinical research or leadership. It is set against this background that serendipitous career opportunities planning is no longer a viable option. Active planning is required. It is important to realise that career choices are not one-off decisions but ongoing lifelong processes.

When you first consider a non-clinical portfolio some colleagues will ask: Why waste all that training? Why reduce and even think of giving up clinical practice? Doctors tend to define themselves as doctors ... meaning the clinician. So if you are considering reducing clinical work to take on a portfolio does that make you less of a doctor? Some may perceive this as a barrier stating that if they reduce clinical hours as compared to their colleagues they will be seen as 'less'. There can be the fear that their reputation as the 'good clinician' will be in some way tarnished or diluted. But again the question to ask yourself is: will I be able, physically and/ or psychologically, to continue doing the same clinical role, on call etc to the same level when I am, say, 40 compared with when I am 60? And a further question is: would I **want** to still be doing what I am doing, full-time clinical, when I am 55 or 60?

Bartle and Thistlewaite (2014) explored the motivations and experience of trainees considering a career in medical education. Six themes emerged:

• Wanting to provide better education
• Personal goals

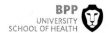

- Expectations/self-direction
- Influence of role models
- Defining one's identity
- Support networks

A barrier to considering such a career pathway was the perception of the need to produce research.

Advantages to portfolio careers

So why seek out a portfolio career in medicine? The answer to this lies in the level of influence you can have with a wider, national role in medical education. There are many benefits. A 35-year career in full-time clinical practice is stressful. A broader portfolio will present new challenges to enable you to develop new skills. This will provide a more varied and richer professional life. It has been suggested that portfolio careers can help to reduce unhappiness in doctors and thus reduce burn out and to improve performance in the range of roles, including the clinical portfolio.

The flexibility potentially afforded by a portfolio career can help a better work–life balance, giving opportunity for family life and also a help in preparing for retirement. Thus, there should be less of a major transition at retirement; it can be phased, retiring from the clinical role and maintaining education for a period of time.

In a medical education role, there is a real opportunity to influence and change the entire healthcare system in which you are working. The common theme running like a golden thread through all of this is – services for patients. In a medical education career portfolio you will in likelihood only be one step away from direct patient care through your direct influence on education and training.

In addition, there are potentially benefits for your employers as encouraging and supporting portfolio careers enhances clinical practice, helps build mutually beneficial partnerships and increases recruitment and retention and improves standards. In the UK these standards from the General Medical Council (GMC) have been made mandatory for every institution that teaches and trains medical students and trainee doctors.

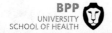

Case study

The undergraduate curriculum in my medical school was fairly traditional in shape: a lot of science in the early years with some patient contact but not integrated in any way. I was working three days a week as a surgeon and two days as a senior lecturer in medical education. I had overall responsibility for teaching across the school. I believed that the curriculum should give the students equal clinical experience and science exposure from day one with the use of problem-based learning. There was so much debate about what problem-based learning was, but as a surgeon I knew that in day to day practice I was faced with 'problems' to solve. So, after two years of working on the plan I was, with the team, able to introduce an integrated experience with a lot of problem-based learning as the main teaching method. The feedback from the first year students was so positive and has subsequently been seen to have better prepared the students for their Foundation Year 1 year. They tell me they feel more confident when faced with a patient problem as a newly qualified doctor.

Summary of what we want in a career

- Variety of interests
- Interesting people
- Satisfaction
- Good company
- Security
- Money
- Chance for development
- Control over what I do
- Using my experience to make decisions
- The amount I earn
- Being with people I like/respect
- Doing a job that is respected by others

Seeking all of the above in one career path is a risky business and spreading your portfolio can help you with all of these.

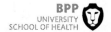

Disadvantages of portfolio careers

With a range of roles there is a risk of overcommitment from both a logistical and psychological point of view. Logistically diary clashes and tension can then leave you unable to contribute at the correct level to either portfolio. There is also the potential for conflict of interest and this will need careful management. A major challenge in one role can spill over into others and as a result the pressure and tension can be generalised.

With interesting additional portfolios there is a risk of loss of interest and hence loss of commitment to the main or original clinical role. You will need to manage multiple employers ('task masters') with rapidly changing agendas. In a medical education career you have to deal with professional and statutory standards, through the Royal Colleges and the regulators.

Career decision-making

In starting to consider a portfolio career there are a number of career decision-making models or tools you can use. A useful one that has been applied to medicine is described by Elton and Reid (2008) in their book *The Roads to Success*. They describe four steps that are useful for you to use to help steer your decision-making and ultimately get you to where you want to be.

1. Self-assessment
2. Explore options
3. Make a decision
4. Implement your plan

1. Self-assessment

Self-assessment is about reflecting. There are a series of questions you will need to ask yourself. These include:

- What is most/least important to you in a career?

- Are these values you hold today likely to change in the future?

- Do you know what your personal strengths and limitations may be and have you sought feedback about these?

- Where do you see yourself in five or ten years' time?

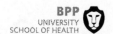

There are a number of simple tasks you can undertake to help you explore and self-assess.

Top tip

Ask ten people you know, all outside of work: what do I do well? You may get ten different answers but the likelihood is you will get ten answers that don't steer you necessarily back to your core clinical role. Those ten answers could help form the basis of a portfolio(s).

Top tip

Look at Box 2.3 where we have described a number of work values. Think about each in turn and against each of them decide for you if they are either:

1. Very important
2. Quite important
3. Not important

Work values

Variety
Geographical location
Money – highly paid
Competitive
Independence in my role
Managing my own time – flexibility
Managing others
Being challenged … 'stretched'

Box 2.3 Work values

Are there lifestyle issues that are important or very important for you? Is geographical location important, being close to family or friends?

How realistic are your initial career plans? Sense check these with friends and family and close colleagues.

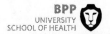

Case study

It all started when I had my second appraisal for revalidation. At that point I had been working in the emergency medicine department for years, ten years I think. It was getting more and more pressured, many patients not needing to be in an ED. All of that. I had a very good appraiser for my second appraisal and she asked me what my career plan was. I had never been asked that before. I had never considered a career plan was needed after I got my consultant post. I could see colleagues mainly in other specialties taking on medical management roles and I always thought that wasn't for me. But the question she asked stuck in my head and then, by chance, I ran into a colleague at a conference. She was now working half time ED and half time for the local Postgraduate Deanery leading on quality issues. This sounded like a very rewarding and challenging role and had taken her out of the ED for half the week, describing it as a lovely balance. This set me thinking. I had always trained trainees but wasn't really aware of career opportunities beyond that.

There are formal methods you can use to self-assess, such as widely used personality inventories such as the Myers-Briggs Type Indicator (MBTI). This is available online and the results should not be used in isolation but just as another set of reflections that you use to steer your thinking.

2. *Explore options*

The case study above is a not uncommon scenario and emphasises the usefulness of using your natural networks. Seek and ask advice about plans that your local medical school or Postgraduate Deanery has in the pipeline. Be clear about all potential career options and any alternatives. Ask yourself:

- Who could you approach to find out more information?
- Are there plans for major innovations in training education – is there a major curriculum revision coming up?
- What role might you have in that?

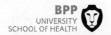

Seek out role models and potential sponsors. What skills do you have? You will have skills and experience you could bring to the table. Look at the careers section of the *British Medical Journal*. Are they advertising jobs you did not know existed or indeed pique your interest? How well do your skills, experience and interests match the roles you aspire to?

Top tip

 What sort of team player are you? All doctors when asked the question 'are you a team player?' will say yes. What they are frequently using as a reference point is Multi-disciplinary Team working. This clinical role is different to the medical education role.

Don't just think about your individual skills. Ask yourself: what sort of team player am I? In any 'new' team what role will or could you play? In a clinical team you will be sure of your role. But what about in a 'new' medical education team?

A useful framework was described by Meredith Belbin (2010) who studied many teams over a period of time and observed that people in teams tend to take up certain different team roles. Understanding team roles has been shown to improve performance of the team and, importantly for you, understanding your role in a medical education team will allow you to develop your skills. Also understanding your role will improve your contribution to the team. Belbin based these roles on observation and it is clear these are just indicators as behaviour and interpersonal style will vary depending on the circumstances.

Belbin identified nine team roles categorised into three groups:

1. Action orientated
2. People orientated
3. Thought orientated

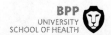

1. Action orientated

i)   Shaper: they challenge the team to improve, are typically extrovert and enjoy shaking up the norms

ii) Implementer: organisers, get the job done, they turn the team ideas into action, work systematically and are well organised

iii) Completer-finisher: they like detail, very conscientious, concerned with meeting deadlines

2. People orientated

i)   Co-ordinator: key focus on tasks, objectives, very organised, they guide the team

ii) Team worker: they are supportive, flexible, diplomatic, help to hold the team together

iii) Resource investigator: they like to explore, investigate the new idea, work with external stakeholders

3. Thought orientated

i)   The plant: the original thinkers, generating new ideas; they bring lateral thinking to the team

ii) Monitor/evaluator: they analyse, weigh evidence, critical thinkers, strategic thinkers

iii) Specialist: they have or want to get specialist skills, technology; for example, an expert in one area

As you move up the medical education ladder in whatever context, undergraduate or postgraduate etc (see Chapters 3, 4 and 5) you will take on formal leadership roles. Each of us will have leadership attributes. The MBTI as discussed above can start to give you clues about yourself that you may or may not be aware of. There are many models of leadership but it is important at the stage of exploring career options to reflect on your leadership style. One model to think about is the opposing autocratic ('do as I say') to the abdicatory ('do what you like') decision-making style. Figure 2.1 shows the spectrum of decision-making style moving from use of authority to giving freedom to staff.

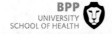
BPP
UNIVERSITY
SCHOOL OF HEALTH

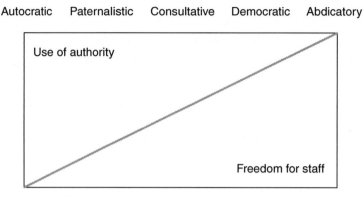

Figure 2.1 The spectrum of decision-making

Your leadership and decision-making style may lie along this continuum. It will or should vary depending on the context but it is worthwhile when exploring specific roles in certain organisations for you to get a sense of that organisation's culture and the bosses' style. Which culture or environment suits you best? This is important. Do you work best in a distributed leadership model where the 'boss' delegates authority and you have or will have a significant amount of autonomy?

• You will have to ask yourself: does a distributed leadership model suit you or do you require more direction and support?

• What is your Plan B if you don't get to follow your 'ideal' route?

Having a plan is good but you will need to be flexible. Always have a Plan B and C. That role that you have always wanted may not come up or be available at the right time for you. Most of the medical educator roles are now much sought after and so the selection process is competitive. You might not be successful ... be flexible and fluid with your plan. It is not failure if you don't achieve Plan A. Similar to any job application you may not be successful the first time. This is not a reason to give up. Applications signal to the employer that you are interested in the role. They may have limited jobs to offer at that time but be clear they will have noticed you and this can be a positive marker for future applications.

Case study

I had always been interested in teaching, mainly medical students in my own specialty and teaching them very specific procedures. The students, as they do, came to me in discrete blocks for four weeks then left and I never saw them again. I began to wonder how what I did fitted into the whole medical school curriculum. I asked the senior tutor about how the year was structured and it didn't really make sense and I couldn't see the joins. It all felt very disjointed. I began to think about taking on more responsibility but really didn't know where to start. The key was asking the right person who then steered me to the lead for the year. The fact I showed an interest lead to me being asked to get involved in the whole curriculum design.

3. Make a decision

If, after exploring, you have a number of competing options you will have to prioritise these. Some useful questions include:

- What are the plus and minus points for each of your career options?

- What kind of working relationships with colleagues do you prefer?

- What effect would your work-style and work–life factors have on opting for one role?

- If you had a choice between opportunities, what would be the critical factors in your decision?

Case study

It was difficult for me to decide on the particular direction I wanted to take. I was involved in the college as an examiner and enjoyed that. I felt I was contributing. I had always had an interest in online learning and had been keen to use technology to improve my own teaching. I felt that we weren't using technology for the benefit of patients or training. I had made a point of learning about coding and programming language and gaining an understanding of how you develop an online platform. At the time I was considering increasing my sessions, if I could, in education. The local Postgraduate Deanery held a training session for educational supervisors in my hospital and at the Question and Answer session I suggested the need for a lead in online learning. Much to my surprise this suggestion was taken up and a job was advertised for an Associate Dean for e-learning. This really was an opportunity as it was the specific area I had been interested in and also my children were still quite young at that point and it suited me to stay locally as opposed to looking at more college roles which would no doubt mean travelling. I applied and was successful.

4. Implement your plan

Once you have made your decision or decided on a number of options for you the next step is planning to get there. Again there are a few key questions you have to ask yourself:

- How up to date is your Curriculum Vitae (CV)?
- What shows 'added value'?
- What have you found out about the likely application process?

Applying for a medical education role is different to applying for a clinical role. Your clinical CV alone will not be appropriate. Look at the advert. Typically there will be a set of essential person specifications. Do not just send in your CV and say 'please see attached'. You will **not** get interviewed. Look in detail at the person specification, provide a paragraph on each, stating that you meet the criteria, and give at least one example of what you have done/ achieved that proves it.

What else do you need to do to prepare yourself?

Volunteer to teach, supervise, lead a workshop. Get noticed. Get a profile. You need to be known if at all possible before applying for medical education roles. You will no doubt be asked the question: 'why are you applying for this role, and why now in your career?'

One very useful question for yourself is:

If you had one minute to sell yourself to an interview panel, what would you say?

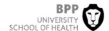

The answer to this question can highlight to you gaps in your experience that may be expected, essential or desirable. Review the essential person specification but also visit the organisation and the department and get a sense of what they are really looking for in the role.

Case study

I had always been interested in medical education and did consider that at some point it would be good to move into this type of role.

I had been College Tutor for a couple of years and had set up a new regional training programme for all the trainees. The feedback was very positive and the exam rate for the membership went to nearly 100%. I added non-clinical skills like management and leadership and these areas were rated very highly by the higher trainees in particular. In order to skill myself up I studied for a Master's in medical education. This made me start to wonder why the Trust didn't have a continuing professional development (CPD) progamme for all doctors in the hospital. We had a lot of non-training grade doctors and 300 consultants and their CPD was driven individually. It really didn't make sense to me. For years within the Trust there had been talk of a lead medical role for education but that's all it appeared to be – talk. Around this time the Trust had a routine GMC visit and the issue of needing a Director of Medical Education type role was flagged. Soon after the Trust advertised for this role and I found that my preparation for the college role helped me to get the Director role. Also my understanding of the postgraduate medical training pathways was very positive.

Planning for that transition of taking on a portfolio will at some point mean letting go of something. The transition from trainee to specialist has been extensively explored and there is recognition that transition to more senior roles requires training and the same applies to portfolio career development.

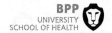

Career map

So what does a typical portfolio career look like? The portfolios can be in parallel or sequential. Most doctors start out with a full-time clinical role, but typically you will also do a little bit of medical student teaching, a little bit of supervising trainees, a little bit of medico legal – just those that come through the NHS. As you move on you get involved in shaping the service, medical management ... so after five years you are doing a little bit of everything, including the original full-time clinical role. There is a significant risk that you will spread yourself too thinly. This cannot go on for the rest of your career (see Chapter 8). There will or should come a time when you have to make conscious career decisions and this will entail stopping something. You will resist this. You will say to yourself: but I like doing x, I don't want to give it up, if I don't do it no one else will, I am the only one who can do this (in the way that I do it or have been doing it). You will have these arguments with yourself.

The career funnel in Figure 2.2 represents the very real risk of not funnelling down and continuing to have a wide range of portfolios that increased your risk of underperforming. This funnelling of your portfolios is an important task and is best planned and not left to chance. If your master plan is to be the next Head of School of Medicine in 'medical school x' then you will have to let go of some of your responsibilities.

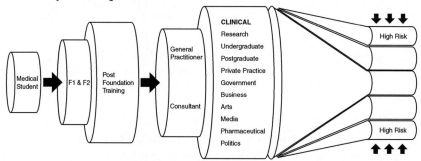

Figure 2.2 The career funnel

As we discuss in other chapters, as you add portfolios or build on one, say, medical education, there does come a point when you will need to drop and let go of more clinical responsibilities.

Chapter summary

Portfolio careers are not new in medicine but are here to stay. This is because a portfolio career can help you to survive, develop your skills, manage your weaknesses better and provide new and fascinating challenges in addition to your clinical career. A medical education portfolio will allow you to have a high level of influence over the education and training of generations of students and doctors.

There is a need for you to plan your career in a flexible manner and a useful framework to use is to self-assess, explore options, come to a decision and devise and implement the plan. You will meet barriers, one of which is the fear of giving up areas of interest to take on new areas. You will have to make those decisions so it is best to do so in a planned fashion.

Key points

- Reflect on where you are in your career and what suits you.
- Plan ahead.
- Prepare yourself to increase your chances of being successful.
- Be flexible – have a Plan B and C.
- Be aware of the need to funnel down in your career pathway.
- Enjoy the challenges.

Useful resources

Myers-Briggs Type Indicator online (www.myersbriggs.org/my-mbti-personality-type/)

References

Bartle, E and Thistlewaite, J. Becoming a medical educator: motivation, socialisation and navigation. *Medical Education* 2014; 14: 110.

Belbin, RM (2010) *Team Roles at Work*. Abingdon: Routledge.

Elton, C and Reid, J (2008) *The Roads to Success*. London: Scribe Publications.

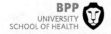

Grey, C. Portfolio Careers. *British Medical Journal* 1996; 313 S2-7057.

Handy, C (1991) *The Age of Unreason*. 2nd edition. London: Century Business.

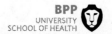

Chapter 3

Undergraduate medical education careers

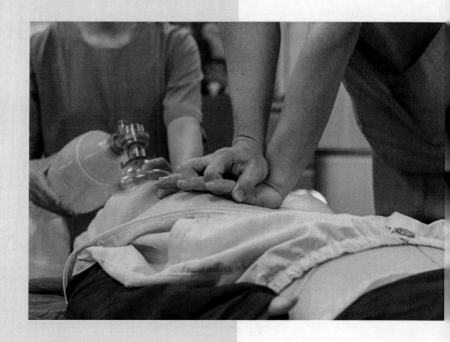

Introduction

A career in medical education opens doors and provides you with many opportunities. If you choose a career pathway in undergraduate (UG) medical education this will usually mean you being employed in a university. In the UK there are 33 medical schools sited in public research universities funded partially by government and currently 2 private medical schools, although this number is on the increase. Medical schools are located in every region in the UK so you have a wide geographical choice.

Medical schools in the UK
Northern Ireland
Queen's University Belfast, Faculty of Medicine and Health Sciences
Wales
Cardiff University, School of Medicine
Swansea University, College of Medicine
Scotland
Aberdeen (University of), School of Medicine
Dundee (University of), Faculty of Medicine, Dentistry and Nursing
Edinburgh (The University of), College of Medicine and Veterinary Medicine
Glasgow (University of), College of Medical, Veterinary and Life Sciences
St Andrews (The University of), Faculty of Medical Sciences
England
East Anglia
Cambridge (University of), School of Clinical Medicine
Norwich Medical School, University of East Anglia
Greater London
Barts and The London School of Medical and Dentistry, Queen Mary, University of London
Imperial College School of Medicine, London
King's College London School of Medicine (at Guy's King's College and St Thomas' Hospital)

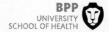

London School of Hygiene and Tropical Medicine (Postgraduate Medical School)
St George's, University of London
University College London, University College Medical School
Midlands
Birmingham (University of), School of Medicine
Keele University, School of Medicine
Leicester (University of), Leicester Medical School
Nottingham (The University of), Faculty of Medicine and Health Sciences
Warwick (University of), Warwick Medical School
North East
Hull York Medical School
Leeds (University of), School of Medicine
Newcastle University Medical School
Sheffield (The University of), School of Medicine
North West
Lancaster University, Faculty of Health and Medicine
Liverpool (University of), Faculty of Health and Life Sciences
Manchester (University of), Faculty of Medicine and Human Sciences
South
Brighton and Sussex Medical School
Oxford (University of), Medical Sciences Division
Southampton (University of), School of Medicine
South West
Bristol (University of), Faculty of Medicine
Exeter (University of), Medical School
Plymouth University Peninsula Schools of Medicine and Dentistry

Table 3.1 Medical schools in the UK

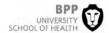

With a school leaver medical school the majority of students come in straight after A Levels and so are 18 years of age. Most of these schools have a 5-year curriculum. Graduate entry medical schools (of which there are 14) typically ask for a 2.1 or above in any subject and offer a 4-year programme. These students are therefore on average older and arguably more mature. They have also perhaps left paid jobs in their fields to pursue a medical career and hence have different views and expectations of a medical degree. So each type of school presents interestingly different challenges.

Typically you will move from your current NHS role more and more into a medical school role and hence university setting. Being in a university setting provides a huge array of challenges but even more opportunities.

Most universities in the UK have a career pathway of either Teaching and Scholarship (T and S) or Teaching and Research (T and R). Most medical education roles will be on the T and S pathway. This is important for progression and promotion up the ladder as described in Figure 3.1. That's not to say if you are on T and S you can't do any research but the focus of your role will be on T and S. The highest-quality medical schools have high-quality teaching underpinned by high-quality research.

Policy drivers in any university worldwide are teaching and research and wrapped around these commonly is innovation and engagement with the local and wider community. The vision or mission statements of most, if not all, medical schools will contain a number of common themes. The first is the quality of teaching and scholarship; the second is high-quality international research.

As an example the home page of University College London (UCL) Medical School states (as of 10 May 2017) the following:

UCL Medical School is committed to excellence in undergraduate and postgraduate education and has a strong reputation for teaching informed by cutting-edge research.

Reflecting the global view Harvard Medical School in Boston, Massachusetts, states (as of 10 May 2017):

Mission. To create and nurture a diverse community of the best people committed to leadership in alleviating human suffering caused by disease.

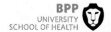

Community values. Harvard Medical School is a community dedicated to excellence and leadership in medicine through education, research and clinical care. We aspire to excellence through a commitment to our community values.

These vision and mission statements are very similar to all medical schools around the globe and give you a sense of the core values of the organisations.

The undergraduate (UG) career pathway

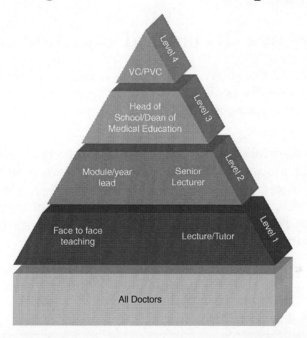

Figure 3.1 The career pathway in undergraduate medical education

As a Clinical Lecturer/Lecturer you will typically be responsible for the day to day delivery of teaching. At this level you are typically a trainee, consultant or General Practitioner (GP) who delivers teaching sessions in your own subject/specialty area.

At a Senior Lecturer level you will deliver some day to day teaching but increasingly have wider responsibilities as an organiser and a module lead and in managing a number of tutors (clinical and non-clinical).

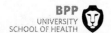

At Reader level you will have more overall responsibility for a theme, eg the assessment strategy, feedback strategy or for example a year lead or programme director.

At Professorial level you have increasing seniority which means increasing responsibility for more areas, functions and outputs; curriculum design is one example.

As you move up the career ladder you will have less face to face responsibilities in teaching but wider influence on more of the entire curriculum.

Drivers in a UG medical education career

In a medical school you will have a range of roles and responsibilities driven by a number of issues. These will give you challenges that will determine your objectives and hence the focus of your thinking and behaviour.

Within a medical school setting, within a university, you will be faced with a number of main drivers. There are a multitude of these but at a strategic level the three main ones are the National Student Survey (NSS), what is currently called the Research Excellence Framework (REF) and the General Medical Council (GMC) standards (GMC, 2015).

The NSS is a high profile survey of mainly final year students in all subjects. The students provide direct, anonymous feedback on a series of questions, essentially asking what it is like to study on their course at that university.

The NSS is high profile, because of it being published in the public domain and it gives potential students and parents of those potential students a clear indicator of current students' views of particular courses. The NSS is currently made up of 23 questions related to the following:

- The teachers on my course
- Assessment and feedback
- Academic support
- Organisational management
- Learning resources
- Personal development
- Overall satisfaction

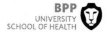

Each student is presented with a range of options from 'definitely agree' to 'not applicable' and also free text boxes where the students can reflect on the positives and negatives.

The NSS is made available to all students through the 'Uni-stats' website so, if you are working in a formal medical education role at whatever level in a medical school, the results on the NSS are a major driver for change in terms of those areas of the curriculum described above.

League tables of medical schools are published by the press, including the Times Good University Guide and the Guardian University League Table. *The Times* uses a complex formula which includes NSS, research quality, entry standards, number of firsts and 2.1s and financial spend on facilities. These are important because students and parents take heed of them. Hence in a medical school these will be issues you will need to take into account.

The other significant driver that is mentioned above is REF. In the UK, REF is the current system for the quality of research of all UK higher education institutions so, depending on your specific role within a medical school, you will have more or less responsibility around REF. For example, within the typical medical education careers described in Figure 3.1 if you are a Dean of Medical Education (DoMe), your main focus will be, in terms of external drivers, the NSS and the GMC standards. If you move into a Head of Medical School (HoMS) role you will be responsible for the quality of teaching as measured through NSS and the GMC but also ultimately responsible for the performance on REF.

Reflecting on this, there is not necessarily a need for you to be a four star leading researcher in medical education in order to move into a HoMS role. Clearly if you have significant research experience this will help, but it is really in essence again back to this principle of building a team around you and therefore within the requirement of REF, as all universities will have a 'REF team'. Your role will be in leading that team.

REF is essentially a process whereby the medical school, as well as all other research-orientated schools, submit their research activity. Currently the submissions to REF remain in 36 areas called units of assessment and so in a medical school the key units of assessment are likely to be:

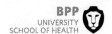

- Clinical medicine
- Public health services and primary care
- Biological sciences

There are currently a total of 36 units which also include physics and mathematical sciences and computer sciences. So it is likely that research teams in your medical school will be working collaboratively with colleagues in other schools and professions all submitting contributions to REF. The importance of REF is that it dictates funding into the organisation; again like NSS, REF results are published and therefore it is extremely important in attracting staff and grants and in the overall reputation of the medical school.

In any medical school in the UK the quality of teaching will need to meet the current GMC standards which now apply to the delivery of all stages of medical education, UG and postgraduate. Extracts for the standards that will impact on your behaviour include the following (these are just examples):

Medical schools (and the universities of which they are a part) manage and control the quality of education leading to the award of their primary medical qualifications. They make sure Local Education Providers (LEPs) appropriately educate their medical students by providing appropriate placements.

Medical schools, postgraduate deaneries and Local Education and Training Boards (LETBs) must have agreements with LEPs to provide education and training to meet the standards. They must have systems and processes to monitor the quality of teaching, support, facilities and learning opportunities on placements, and must respond when standards are not being met.

Medical schools must have one or more doctors at the school who oversee medical students' educational progression. They must have one or more doctors at each LEP who co-ordinate training of medical students, supervise their activities, and make sure these activities are of educational value.

Medical schools (and the universities of which they are a part) must have a process to make sure that only those medical students who are fit to practise as doctors are permitted to graduate with a primary medical qualification. Medical students who do not meet the outcomes for graduates or who are not fit to practise must not be allowed to graduate with a medical degree or continue on a medical programme. Universities must make sure that their regulations allow compliance by medical schools with GMC requirements with respect to primary medical qualifications. Medical schools must investigate and take action when there are concerns about the fitness of medical students to practise, in line with GMC guidance. Doctors in training who do not satisfactorily complete a programme for provisionally registered doctors must not be signed off to apply for full registration with the GMC.

These extracts from the GMC's current standards give a flavour of the roles and responsibilities you will need to focus on in a medical education role in a medical school. As HoMS, or delegated to a DoMe, you are directly accountable to the GMC for the quality of all aspects of the learning experience of students.

You will therefore spend a lot of time developing processes and teams to ensure the following challenges are met.

Curriculum design: The trend in most medical schools is to have early exposure to patient contact and an integrated curriculum where science is embedded in clinical learning and bedside learning.

The school's teaching strategy will need to align with the ethos of the curriculum, be it problem-based learning for example. What that may mean in practice is implementing revisions of the curriculum, redirecting activities of certain staff, negotiating and leading change. So you will need to not only understand the theory and practice of education principles but also manage and lead people. A medical education career is about people.

Increasing student numbers: In any medical school a major source of income to fund teaching posts comes from the number of students on the programme and international students attract more money.

Admissions policy: You will need a robust and GMC-agreed admissions process. There is increasing recognition of the need for admissions to facilitate widening access and diversity. Indeed there is a government directive to demonstrate how each school is achieving this. You will link very closely with the Universities and Colleges Admissions Service.

Links with NHS: You will be required to keep abreast of any innovations in NHS service delivery. In recent years there has been

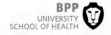

a policy shift leading to a blurring of boundaries between primary and secondary care, with more 'secondary care' services moving into the community. Students will therefore need more placements in the community. These can be more difficult to organise and manage logistically and more expensive.

Training the trainers: In the UK the GMC has set out standards for recognition (at medical school level) for lead co-ordinators of UG training and any doctor responsible for overseeing students' educational process. In reality this means that if you have dedicated sessions and specific responsibilities you will need to meet those standards. If responsible for the medical school's recognition of trainers you will need to ensure a process is in place to train and record the continuing professional development of your tutors, lecturers and senior lecturers.

Multidisciplinary teaching: Within the NHS there is now a focus on Multi-disciplinary Teams at the hub of patient care and hence a focus on multiprofessional learning. This will increasingly need to be reflected in the medical UG curricula. There are risks here for you in a DoMe or HoMS role in that, with workforce developments such as Physician Associates and increased numbers of Advanced Nurse Practitioners in a number of clinical areas, capacity for medical students to gain exposure to certain diseases, syndromes or procedures may be at risk and will be part of what the GMC inspection visits will closely monitor.

Assessment strategy: This is a key issue for you as the GMC will focus on it. How do you assess students' progress and ensure the quality of teaching and learning?

Support for students: This is a vital element. You will need a process for early identification of students underperforming. Underperformance has many causes and students will need a range of support services they can access. Having systems in place to ensure that students are resilient and recognise the importance of their own wellbeing is very important. These support systems link into fitness to practise questions that will arise and you will have to manage these on a day to day basis.

Managing the budget: Financial accountability is central to more senior roles, although in most medical schools this will be devolved across and/or down the organisation but you will need to acquire the skills to manage a budget. This is again an example of how important a team is around you, so you can call on the expertise of a competent Director of Finance or equivalent.

Level 1

Wherever you are on the medical career pathway you will undoubtedly teach. Most, if not all, doctors will teach. This is Level 1 (see Figure 3.1). So as a GP, consultant or Staff and Associate Specialist (SAS) doctor, medical student or trainee you will be working with other colleagues who have less experience and less confidence in certain tasks or procedures. If you are the 'teacher' this will not necessarily take place in a formal classroom scenario, but on the ward or in outpatients. You may show a colleague how to do something, or supervise them briefly and provide an encouraging word. This is the backbone of learning in an NHS setting. This culture of sharing skills and knowledge is a major strength in health. This informal teaching is a central role for any doctor and was set within the original Hippocratic Oath and in more modern versions:

> *I will respect the hard-won scientific gains of those physicians in whose steps I walk, and gladly share such knowledge as is mine with those who are to follow.*

Sometimes this level of teaching isn't referred to as teaching. It's called 'showing the ropes' or 'explaining how the ward works'.

Case study

As a Staff Grade doctor I'm never sure at what point in the day I will teach. Well, sometimes it's not teaching in a classroom but showing students how to examine patients when we are in clinic. So is that instruction? An example is that every six months or so we may or may not have students on placement in the department doing their projects. They are with us, if they choose obstetrics for six weeks full time. The students have a specific project but generally are keen to attend theatre and outpatients and I will show them how to suture and get them to assist. I will, I guess, also talk to them about a career in Obstetrics, get them to report on scans and have a go at ultrasound scans. I am never that sure if what I'm covering is in the curriculum but I know it's all important to do the job day to day.

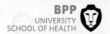

Case study

As a final year surgical trainee I have spent the last three months in the emergency department mainly looking after major trauma. On a day to day basis there are medical students on placement, usually for four to six weeks at a time, and in the last lot a few of them were clearly lacking confidence in suturing. I spent some time with them supervising, helping out and showing them different sutures and knots that they can use. This is all part and parcel of actually being a clinician as I wouldn't have the skills I have today without those trainees and consultants more experienced taking time to teach me.

So at Level 1 teaching you will typically be teaching on the hoof, in the workplace and with one to two learners. As a result, as the teacher you will usually get immediate feedback from the learners. This positive feedback does provide you with instant satisfaction and helps you to feel valued in the role. So you have to want to teach and see it as an integral part of your day to day work.

Case study

A day in the life of a Clinical Lecturer

This day was fairly typical in that I was on a non-clinical day from my clinical training in psychiatry. So within my job plan I have a Thursday and Friday where I am responsible for overseeing the delivery of Year 4 psychological medicine teaching. There are cohorts of medical students that come on a four to six week block.

8:30am. I met up with the undergrad administrator who I work very closely with and we checked that the programme for today was accurate and that the two additional lecturers and facilitators had confirmed that they were attending. We then checked the three seminar rooms that we were going to use for the teaching. The administrator ensured all of the technology and laptops were working. I quickly flicked through my introductory PowerPoint of six slides, which set the scene for the day. Within this I had already spent some time writing out the specific objectives for the day which were essentially around ensuring that the students understood the concepts of risk assessment and were increasingly confident in risk assessment with a patient who was suicidal.

8:55am. The students started to arrive. I was aware that a couple of the students had difficulty with transport from a number of the hospital sites. A few of the students asked to see me separately, and I took them to a separate office and asked them to tell me about their difficulties. In essence they were describing that the school minibus hadn't turned up at the pre-planned time and venue and they were left to then order taxis. This had been an ongoing problem in the medical school and I made a note to myself that I needed to discuss this with the new administrator, but also assure the students that I would do something about it and again reiterated that it wasn't their role to organise taxis and that they should have phoned the administrator on site, who would have been able to organise those taxis for them as the students shouldn't have been out of pocket. The students appeared reasonably satisfied with that approach and I also took the opportunity in this ten minutes just to check and ask them how they were getting on with their studies and how they felt about working in psychiatry. I was basically taking the opportunity of getting informal feedback on their programmes so far.

9:35am. After covering the objectives for the day we had a 10–15 minute question and answer session. I purposefully left this extremely open. There were no significant issues but I was aware that previous cohorts had been somewhat apprehensive about assessing suicide risk and I assured them that the training that they would get would enable them to feel more confident. I explained to them that we would be using actors who had been given a very specific brief and were extremely well trained and experienced in this and it wasn't an assessment throughout the day of their skills, it was an opportunity for them to practise in a very safe environment.

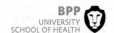

10:00am. All the sessions started with two consultant tutors helping me out. We had 3 rooms but 15 students so the students were split into groups. One of them interviewed the mock patient while the other five or six observed and were given an assessment sheet. So this session went on until 11:30am when we had a break for coffee, another opportunity to network with the students, not just checking how they were getting on academically but also giving them the opportunity to ask us any questions about any aspect of their learning – not just things that I was directly responsible for but if there were any wider issues. We then restarted, finishing at 12:45pm for a 45-minute lunch break. The students went off to the canteen and I planned within the programme to spend 10 or 15 minutes with the two psychiatrists, the actors and the administrators just to have an informal debrief on any particular issues that we needed to deal with.

2:00pm. We restarted the sessions and finished at 4:25pm. I thanked the actors and lecturers and got the students together in another room. I asked them how they felt about the session and how it went. In addition, I made sure that we put out on the desks formal evaluation forms which we were very clear within the curriculum should be anonymised but obviously at that point the students were keen to put their names to the feedback. I saw this as a very positive aspect that they clearly felt safe to give the feedback as they can feel quite vulnerable.

So in summary Level 1 teaching/instructing is where you directly deliver teaching to the learners. That is your level of responsibility. You may or may not be au fait with the details in the medical students' curriculum. At this level you are not responsible for the aims or objectives, or for the delivery of anything wider than what you have taught them.

In the UG career pathway all doctors, GPs, SAS, consultants and trainees would be expected to engage in this level of teaching and this is the starting point for a UG career. Within the UG career ladder you may or may not have any teaching recognised or an honorary title.

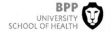

Level 2

At the next level (which we refer to as Level 2) you start to take on wider responsibilities. Typically you move from informal ad hoc teaching to more formal, eg in the classroom teaching a cohort of student nurses or medical students. This more formal learning starts to closely map to specific objectives that the learners have in their curricula.

Case study

It was only when I took on responsibility for the delivery of my own specialty teaching in the school that I realised how complex the curriculum was. Up to that point I naively thought that the students should have to learn everything about my own specialty (Paediatrics) and I was often vocal, insisting that they need more exposure to child health. Getting more involved I realised that the five years is a busy curriculum and the students are under an enormous amount of pressure having to cover so much clinical work/areas. It did give me a fresh perspective on where Paediatrics teaching was in the curriculum and my thinking started to shift to the need for a more integrated approach as when the same students were on the ED block they obviously had a lot of exposure to Paediatrics, although it wasn't badged as Paeds.

So with Level 2 you will be delivering direct one to one and group teaching but in addition you will get involved in designing a specific bit of the curriculum. This could entail being responsible for a particular specialty-based module or block. You will input into the objectives and the teaching methods used to achieve those objectives, for example small group work, simulation or a mixed approach. You will be part of a team that looks at the assessment strategy for the year that the module is in. You will also typically be responsible for managing and leading a small number of colleagues who deliver the module or block. These could be delivering face to face teaching or online. You will still deliver face to face teaching yourself but moving along a continuum. Although you are still delivering teaching directly, there is slightly less of that and more emphasis on organising and leading and supporting others. So that immediate satisfaction you get from students whom you teach is less acutely experienced.

Case study

I had been teaching medical students on the psychiatry block for a number of years. They arrived in blocks of six weeks and I usually taught psychpharmacology. I became more interested in teaching and when the Honorary Senior Lecturer retired I was encouraged to apply for the role. The main difference was that I had to organise the six-week block based on the objectives and looking at the feedback forms from past groups of students. I also had to manage a half-time admin person and this was new to me so there was a learning curve. I was still delivering face to face teaching but more of my time was spent organising the block. I was still getting positive feedback but the balance of my time was shifting towards managing and leading the teaching. As a result I started to become involved in the school-wide group that looked across the specialty-based blocks and was keen to look at common objectives that we as a group of tutors across specialties could deliver in an integrated way. So the biggest change was having to manage and lead colleagues in my specialty, particularly when there were issues with teaching approaches and other logistical issues.

So at Level 2 typically you would be at Lecturer or Senior Lecturer level, usually still full-time clinical or with one or two sessions within the medical school but starting down the medical education portfolio career pathway. You may be responsible for the delivery of teaching in your own specialty or a theme such as communication skills. Now for some doctors that is as far as it goes and they are happy to contribute at that level and that is great.

Level 3

At this level you are now the DoMe or HoMS. As the latter you are essentially the Chief Executive Officer (CEO) of the organisation and your role is leadership. You now lead and manage the senior team in the school who manage the educators/lecturers. It is at this point that your leadership style and your people management skills are key. So as you have moved up the career ladder or across the

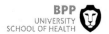

bridge in Generation Y terms you now have less and less direct teaching responsibilities, therefore perhaps less opportunity for immediate positive feedback; you have to look to the longer game but have significantly higher levels of influence. So, with less direct teaching you will have generally less opportunity for direct immediate feedback but a higher level of influence on a larger number of learners – therefore it's a trade-off.

What is expected of you?

When applying for substantive medical education roles at Level 3, so for example a DoMe, it is useful to start to look at adverts for these types of posts and obtain the job descriptions. This is important because you will see that in general the main functions will be described within the job descriptions and they typically follow the following format:

1. Your role will be to oversee the strategic enhancement development of UG medical teaching and learning within the medical school.

2. You will be responsible for ensuring that all activities map to the university's wider strategic aims and mission objectives.

3. You will be expected to apply strategic leadership of UG teaching within the medical school and develop opportunities and be innovative around those developments for all students.

4. You will provide strategic leadership for all aspects of recruitment and selection into the medical school and policies to support the students, both academically and pastorally.

5. You will develop education strategies to meet the increasing demands of the NHS and initiate policies aimed at promoting the requirements of the NHS such as clinical governing and professionalism within the UG curriculum.

6. You will lead, supervise and support the development of the UG's medical team and Faculty, including ensuring that all teachers, lecturers are meeting the regulatory standards for lecturer/trainer recognition.

7. You will embody excellence in research-informed and research-driven teaching, and inspire others to do the same.

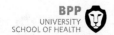

There will also be a person specification, typically including:

1. PG certificate in medical/dental education or equivalent (member of higher education academy, academy of medical educators or similar recognised professional educator body (see Chapter 6 for qualifications).

2. Substantial (minimum x years) and significant teaching experience at UG or PG level, demonstrating teaching innovation in course design and delivery. Even if a post is in the UG arena experience in PG is typically 'counted' and held to be of equal standing.

3. Substantial clinical (min of x years) experience and the ability if no longer clinically active to keep up to date.

4. Established reputation for teaching excellence, educational innovation and learner empowerment/enablement, within the field of science or medicine or dentistry.

5. Proven ability to adapt to the changing environments of the higher education community.

6. Proven exceptional strategic leadership ability in a higher education context.

7. Experience of leading large-scale programme development with the ability to lead and manage change through inspiring and motivating others (give an example here).

8. Evidence of contribution to scholarship, for example, through research leading to the authorship of books/textbooks, editorship of journals or journal articles, development/design of teaching materials or successful applications for external funding for learning developments.

9. A commitment to the centrality of high quality patient care as the end product of medical education.

Top tip

 As with any interview: rehearse, prepare, read, discuss (see Chapter 2). Interviews for medical education roles are not the same as those you will be used to when applying for clinical roles.

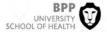

Now, when initially looking at these main functions, it can be difficult to understand how you could possibly deliver against such broad aims, but typically within a university setting you will have an annual appraisal, with possibly six-monthly reviews and be given specific objectives in terms of, for example, curriculum design, curriculum revision, embedding problem-based learning and helping to support academic and pastoral support for medical students.

So at Level 3 you will have overall responsibility for all activities within the medical school. For the two strands of teaching and research, again the key is a good team. At this level there are of course many leadership styles but in an organisation as complex as the average medical school you are required to be the strategic lead, setting the direction of travel. Your role is to have a clear sense of the direction of travel of the big ticket issues and supporting the team around you (see Chapter 8). In the UK most HoMS will be outward-facing CEO-type roles and networking at a UK and international level is a very important component of the role.

At a UK level you will as a HoMS be a member of the Medical Schools Council. This is a UK-wide body representing the interests and ambitions of UK medical schools. There will be opportunities to expand your role and influence into the GMC, advising Government and taking on UK lead roles in certain areas.

At a practical level you will lead the team when the regulators visit to quality assure all aspects of the teaching. The outcome of GMC visits is important as these are published on their website. The GMC may undertake a themed visit to your region or a specific routine cycle of visits to medical schools and PG Deaneries (or equivalent) in a region. So it is important that strategically you have meaningful working relationships with your local PG Deanery.

Case study

A day in the life of a Head of Medical School

8:30am. I had a pre-meeting for the new post of Professor in Emergency Medicine. I was chairing the interview panel on behalf of the Vice Chancellor. This was a sensitive matter as the local NHS Trust was part funding the new post and there was likely to be a difference of opinion about the candidates. As it was, my preferred candidate was clearly more suited to the role and all parties were happy. A good result.

11:00am. Next was a meeting with HR regarding a reorganisation I had triggered attempting to ensure that those staff on a T and R were producing or had the potential to produce high-quality research and those on T and S were delivering high-quality teaching and were qualified teachers.

2:00pm. This was a 20-minute meeting to discuss the details of next year's graduation and in particular identifying appropriate individuals who could be put forward to the university's governing body to be awarded an Honorary Fellowship.

3:30pm. Next was a meeting with student reps from each of the years to listen to any feedback they have for me. These were regular monthly meetings and were generally very constructive. This was in large part because of the high calibre of the reps. The three suggestions they came up with had been discussed by some of the faculty team. Transport between hospital sites when on clinical placements was a key one. I agreed that we would purchase a minibus.

5:00pm. My final meeting of the day was with the Vice Chancellor and CEO of our neighbouring NHS Trust about funding for additional Professors in key research themes. I had wanted ten new chairs and these negotiations had been going on for six months. We all agreed that the Professors for Genetics and Psychiatry were priorities for all of us so we were able to agree. The Trust was happy as we agreed 50/50 funding resulting in more support for the clinical services.

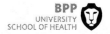

So as a HoMS you will focus on NSS, GMC, standards, welfare of the students, wellbeing, training your staff, money, politics and compromise. You will not necessarily be popular in this role. It is not a popularity contest! You will be faced with difficult and complex decisions, and you have to make a call on them.

In your journey through these 'artificial levels', people are key. Medical education is a people business. In your career pathway seek out support mentors. You will be inspired by people, by innovators. You will also inspire those around you. You should not underestimate your influence on those around you as a role model.

There are a range of further opportunities that arise out of a UG medical education career. Within a university setting there are career opportunities beyond HoMS into, for example, a Pro Vice Chancellor role for a health college, then Deputy Vice Chancellor and the Vice Chancellor. These are all possible as the skills you will acquire on your journey will be transferable.

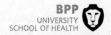

Chapter summary

Careers in UG medical education typically sit with universities and as you move along this career pathway you can have increasing levels of responsibility and influence. Along the way you will acquire skills and knowledge that are transferable.

Key points

- For UG medical education careers you are usually employed in a university setting.

- There are a wide range and diversity of medical schools.

- You will have influence at pivotal times in a doctor's career.

- There is a clear career pathway.

Useful resources

Medical Schools Council site: www.medschools.ac.uk/AboutUs/Pages/default.aspx

National Student Survey site: www.thestudentsurvey.com

Research Excellence Framework site: www.ref.ac.uk

References

General Medical Council (2015) *Promoting Excellence: Standards for Medical Education and Training*. [Online]. Available at: www.gmc-uk.org/education/standards.asp [Accessed 21 June 2017].

General Medical Council (2012) *Recognising and Approving Trainers: the Implementation Plan*. [Online]. Available at: www.gmc-uk.org/Approving_trainers_implementation_plan_Aug_12.pdf_56452109.pdf [Accessed 21 June 2017].

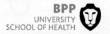

Chapter 4

Postgraduate education careers

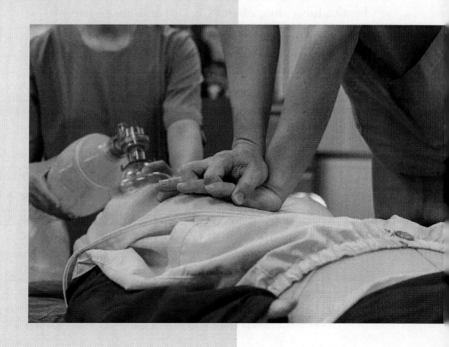

Chapter 4

Introduction

There are numerous jobs in the postgraduate arena for anyone looking to develop their educational career. Many of these jobs will obviously reside within the local Postgraduate Deanery or Local Education and Training Boards (LETBs) in England. There are currently a total of 19 Deaneries or similar organisations across the UK.

Postgraduate Deaneries and LETBs across the UK
Defence Postgraduate Medical Deanery
Health Education East Midlands
Health Education East of England
Health Education England working across Kent, Surrey and Sussex
Health Education England working across West Midlands
Health Education England working across Yorkshire and the Humber
Health Education North Central and East London
Heath Education North East
Health Education North West
Health Education North West London
Health Education South London
Health Education South West
Health Education Thames Valley
Health Education Wessex
Northern Ireland Medical and Dental Training Agency
Scotland Deanery
Wales Deanery

Table 4.1 Postgraduate Deaneries and LETBs across the UK

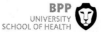

Postgraduate medical education roles can involve anything from one to two sessions per week right up to full-time work as a senior member of the Deanery team. A quick glance at any Deanery website will show the full range of work undertaken by the Deanery and therefore the roles that need filling to achieve this.

The Postgraduate Deanery is responsible for the training in secondary care and vocational training in General Practice. It is also responsible for dental training and training the wider dental Multi-disciplinary Team. Indeed many Deaneries are focused not solely on doctor or dental trainees but on the whole multiprofessional healthcare community.

Supporting recruitment to training places also remains the responsibility of the Deanery as does the quality management of training within the geographical patch. These roles are very important, as ensuring there are enough trainees in the system and levels of vacancies in training programmes can become highly politicised. The Deanery also answers directly to the General Medical Council (GMC) for its quality management processes and employs doctors in leading roles for these tasks.

Many of the roles within the Deanery may be familiar to you and Figure 4.1 shows an example of a typical Deanery organisational design.

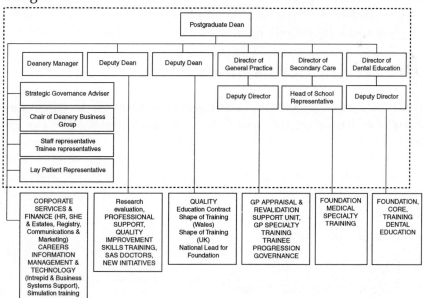

Figure 4.1 Organisational chart of a Deanery as an example

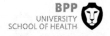

The postgraduate career pathway

So as a General Practitioner (GP) or consultant your first formal medical education role in the postgraduate arena is likely to be in the role of GP trainer or Educational Supervisor (ES). These are roles formally recognised by the GMC. The GMC's definition of ES in secondary care will give you a flavour of what is expected:

> *An Educational Supervisor is defined as – a trainer who is selected and appropriately trained to be responsible for the overall supervision and management of a trainee's trajectory of learning and educational progress during a placement or series of placements. Every trainee must have a named educational supervisor. The educational supervisor helps the trainee to plan their training and achieve agreed learning outcomes. He or she is responsible for the educational agreement and for bringing together all relevant evidence to form a summative judgement at the end of the placement or series of placements.*

(GMC website as of 10 May 2017)

In these roles you will commit to undertaking training relevant to the role, to developing your skills and competencies and to engaging in supporting activities such as recruitment to training grade posts and participation in Annual Review of Competency Progression (ARCP) panels. As an ES or GP trainer you are a part of your specialty school, each of which sits in the local Deanery.

The GP trainer as an example

A GP trainer is typically appointed by the Deanery to teach and train one doctor on the vocational training scheme. The doctor will be assigned to the practice of the trainer and undertake surgeries and visits at a pace determined by their experience and in discussion with the trainer. It is important to realise that the whole practice has to be considered a training practice and meet defined standards such as:

- Written protocols
- Fully summarised notes
- Repeat prescribing protocols
- Manageable workload

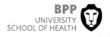

- Offering a wide range of services
- Protected time available for the trainer to fulfil the role
- A commitment from everyone in the practice to have a good educational environment conducive to learning and teaching

The trainer needs to have time to fulfil the role and will be required to have protected teaching time every week. This usually involves one session per week where they can get together with the trainee for a tutorial. The content of this can vary from ensuring the delivery of the curriculum to hot topics and discussion of any issues that have come up that week. The trainer is responsible for supporting the trainee in preparation for the ARCP process and should be reviewing the trainee's portfolio to ensure progress during the year.

The trainer will also be the first port of call for the trainee and will review their surgery and visiting notes. Depending on the vocational training scheme the experience of the trainee can be variable. They can arrive straight out of the Foundation Programme or be in practice for the last year of the training scheme. It is necessary to tailor the programme (and indeed the expectations of the staff) to the actual stage of their training. Essential skills for the trainer are in one to one teaching, giving feedback and career advice and generally supporting the trainee.

The local GP Training Scheme will usually run a trainers group, which generally meets monthly. This is a support group for the trainers and an opportunity to discuss issues related to training and the progress of the trainees themselves. Continuing professional development (CPD) is an important part of being a trainer and the Regional Adviser for GP will organise courses throughout the year to help keep the trainers up to date.

Approval for undertaking the role of a trainer is usually in three-year cycles. At the end of that time there will be a visit from representatives of the Deanery regional GP team. They will want to know that the practice is still committed to training and that the systems and protocols continue to be up to date. They will interview all relevant staff, the partners, the trainee and indeed the trainer. The trainer will also be asked to video a recent surgery so again the visitors can assure themselves that the trainer is practising medicine to the highest standards.

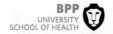

Following the visit recommendations will be made about the practice keeping its training status and any suggestions for further improvement. There is currently a trainers grant that the practice receives and, while this may not be a large sum of money for the responsibility of training, the practice does benefit from having a trainee and clearly from maintaining the highest standards of patient care commensurate with its training status. GP trainers can find the one to one teaching aspect richly rewarding as the trainee develops in the role.

Training Programme Director

As you obtain more experience as a General Practice trainer or ES you may want to take on wider responsibilities such as a Training Programme Director (TPD) or Course Organiser in General Practice.

As TPD you will have responsibilities for all aspects of the training programme in a geographical patch. A sample of the responsibilities you might have as TPD include the following:

- Programme management
  - To manage the placement of new and existing trainees on the rotation
  - To work with local educators to manage and quality control training within all training units in the area
  - To validate training posts within the Local Education Providers (LEPs) on an annual basis, to ensure the training programme meets the requirements of the GMC and Gold Guide
  - To ensure that all trainees have access to suitable training which will allow them the opportunity to achieve the requirements for satisfactory completion of their training
- Appraisal and assessment
  - To monitor trainee progress and performance at regular intervals through liaison with College Tutors and the Professional Support Lead as well as the ARCP process
  - To initiate remedial support for any trainee who experiences difficulty, working with the Professional Support Lead and the Professional Support Unit as required
  - To lead and participate in ARCP panels

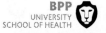

- Trainee support
  - To work with the Professional Support Unit to ensure trainees receive appropriate support where required
  - To arrange placements for trainees with special educational needs where necessary
  - To advise trainees on processes for inter-Deanery transfers, out of programme experience etc

Other responsibilities include development of the programme, recruitment, quality management and careers guidance. So, as a TPD you can have a significant level of influence on the wider training agenda at the same time as continuing regular contact with trainees in your specialty.

Specific specialty school portfolios

The next step on from a TPD role in a postgraduate medical education career could be to take on a lead role in your specialty school such as lead for careers, quality management, less than full time or education initiatives. There are a varied range of opportunities with a different emphasis across all Deaneries. So a good starting point is to look at your local Deanery's website. Network with colleagues. Seek opportunities.

These portfolios may then lead you to take on wider responsibility not just within your specialty school but also across the Deanery. These roles are typically at Associate Dean level with a formal commitment to between one and four sessions per week.

Examples of wider Deanery roles

1. Quality lead
2. Performance support
3. Careers guidance
4. Special projects/initiatives

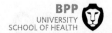

1. **Quality lead**

   The quality management of training is the single most important role that a Deanery fulfils. The Deanery quality lead will be responsible for the following:

   - Organising the quality visits to every educational provider
   - Analysing the GMC trainee and trainer survey returns
   - Communicating the survey results to Health Boards/Trusts and departments
   - Flagging issues that are raised for further investigation
   - In-depth review of any issues related to bullying or harassment
   - Point of contact for training issues for LEPs
   - Answering queries in regard to quality of training issues to external bodies
   - Making recommendations to the Dean in regard to removal of trainees

   These are just some of the functions that the quality lead would have to undertake which places them firmly at the centre of the quality of training agenda.

2. **Performance support**

   All Deaneries have a team that looks after the interests of those doctors who, for whatever reason, are having difficulties in progressing in their training programme. This could be related to ill health, examination failure, wrong career choice, disciplinary procedures or referral to the GMC. The role of the lead is to help the trainee and make the necessary referral to occupational health counselling services or just to support them through the particular issues that they are facing. The lead can be seen as an 'honest broker' in these cases as they are not the direct employer and have access to more support services. The various performance leads in every Deanery meet at a UK-wide level to discuss the services they offer and the support available. This exchange of ideas has proved valuable in ensuring a uniform approach across the UK to the support trainees can expect.

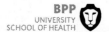

The lead may well also have to make recommendations that the individual should be removed from training and will have had to have made a fully documented case for this to happen. On the positive side, the vast majority of trainees who have difficulties are able to return to their normal training programme after accessing appropriate support.

3. **Careers guidance**

Another aspect of the Deanery team will involve individuals who are there to offer career guidance to trainees. This involves ensuring that information is available on the Deanery website about career choices and how to get one to one help. Attendance at the career fairs and giving talks to the local medical school are favoured options. It is essential to know what other sources of information are available and there is a national website which is kept up to date. The job can also involve running courses on preparation of CVs, interview techniques and what to expect as a new consultant or GP. There is no specific qualification required for this role though some choose to undertake a Master's degree in career guidance.

4. **Special projects/initiatives**

There is another aspect of the Deanery role that looks to innovate and look wider at what can be offered to the training programmes. These can be one-off short-term projects or just additions to the portfolios of senior Deanery team members. A typical list of activities could look like:

- Smartphone technology by the bedside
- Resilience training
- Leadership training
- Quality improvement projects
- Trainer development
- Simulation-based training projects
- Deanery awards and prizes for educational developments
- Mobile apps for CPD

One very positive aspect to these initiatives is that they can be responsive to demand, invariably are led by an enthusiastic person, give benefit to the work and reputation of the Deanery and are responsive to financial pressures.

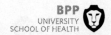

Some of these so-called non-clinical skills such as those under the banner of leadership or quality improvement will be increasingly important and therefore are likely to generate new roles and career opportunities in Deaneries. These areas have been described in the GMC's generic professional capabilities, the themes of which are covered in Chapter 7.

Head of Specialty School

The model of leads for each of the specialty schools has gone under numerous revisions over the last few years. These individuals are appointed to give direct feedback and advice on all issues related to training and recruitment within the specialty to the Deanery. A pathway into these roles, although not always, includes previous experience as a TPD or College Tutor.

Collectively Heads of Specialty Schools (HoSS) meet with the wider Deanery team on a regular basis to discuss issues, problems, any changes to standards or curriculum, the ARCP process, examination results and Trust/Heath Board specific issues that the Deanery may need to be aware of and act on. They are the person who will liaise with Clinical Tutors and ESs when a trainee is in difficulty in the first instance. They may well be able to resolve the issue locally with a low-key approach. However, they will be aware of and act according to the Deanery protocol for quality issues and can therefore escalate according to the severity of the issue. A HoSS will check that the trainees in the specialty are receiving the necessary protected teaching time, study leave, outpatient attendance and theatre time as appropriate and again signal to the Deanery if issues are arising.

The usual number of sessions for this role is between two and four (paid at the sessional rate the doctor is currently on) but for the larger specialties it can be more depending on the overall time commitment required. So with these roles there is still usually a significant clinical commitment but you will be funnelling into a most specialised portfolio career.

This job gives a good insight into the wider running of the specialty and the quality agenda and individual issues with trainees and ESs. It also offers direct links into the senior Deanery team and all the support that that entails.

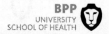

Foundation School Director

In the UK the Foundation Programme has been in place since 2006 and each LETB and Deanery has a Foundation School Director to oversee the programme. This role covers the following:

- Recruitment to the Foundation Year 1 jobs and matching to the Foundation Year 2 jobs

- Recruiting ESs

- Balancing the educational content of the jobs across the two years

- Developing and reviewing the academic foundation programmes

- Recruiting to the academic foundation programmes

- Setting up centres for the situational judgement tests (ranking exam for foundation placements)

- Placing the students according to their rank and preferences

- Setting up the ARCP panels and appeals

- Dealing with doctors failing to progess

- Ensuring adherence to Deanery quality standards

- Considering applications for special circumstances, inter-Deanery transfers and reasonable adjustments to the workplace

- Placing students with special needs in more supportive environments

- Ensuring the sign-off for full registration and Year 2 paperwork is completed in a timely fashion

As can be seen, this is an involved job with a major administrative burden but does form the bridge between the medical school and the first years in specialty or GP training.

There has been a focus on increasing the number of community placements in the programme and this clearly has a knock-on effect to service provision in secondary care. This need to be negotiated and the director is well placed to undertake this role. The number and placements of the academic programmes also need to be thought through as again they are important to link those who wish to have an academic career going forward.

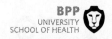

The other major issue that has occurred in the UK Foundation Programme is that of undersubscription to the programme. This has happened over the last several years and can leave gaps in the programme which are hard to fill at the last moment. The director will have to decide how best to place those that have applied to their school. However, the matter is complicated by the fact that the students give a preference for a particular geographical area and that usually means the less popular areas are always left short of trainees. Difficult decisions have to be made by the director in conjunction with the receiving Health Boards/Trusts. The advent of the new private medical school and the increase in medical school numbers (1,500) in England may well mean that this is a thing of the past but will still need managing in the interim. The director will clearly need support from the Deanery team on such issues.

Director of General Practice

Every Deanery and LETB has a GP Director who oversees all issues pertaining to General Practice in the locality. The director answers directly to the Postgraduate Dean and is a member of the senior Deanery team. The job is predominantly the business of the GP section and man management of the staff and extended staff employed in education-related jobs across the patch. Many of the current GP Directors still practise part time as GPs so few are actually full time in the role. However, they will invariably be doing usually six to eight sessions in the role.

The common pathway to be the GP Director is to have come up 'through the ranks' from GP trainer to Course Organiser, Regional Adviser and on to the director post. This progression will give you a very solid understanding of the roles and responsibilities of those on your team and a good insight into what can be achieved with the available resources. Taking meetings could be considered the mainstay of the role and would include the following:

- Input into senior Deanery team and the overall strategic direction of the Deanery

- Meeting with own senior GP team

- Meeting with finance director for regular updates on spending

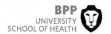

- Recruitment and retention of GP trainees and updates on recruitment figures
- Review of the ARCP processes
- Dealing with trainees in difficulty
- Inter-Deanery transfers
- Dealing with problems in training practices
- Speaking at regional away days for trainers
- Staff recruitment and retention issues

The GP Director will also be a member of the Committee of General Practice Education Directors. This is where all the GP Directors and many of their deputies meet to discuss issues at a UK-wide level. It is a supportive organisation and provides excellent networking opportunities. It also provides the focus for discussions that effect recruitment and retention and the movement of GPs from one Deanery to another. It provides the regulator (GMC) with an opportunity to update all directors on any change to the standards required and training environment.

The Director role can also be a stepping-stone to becoming a Postgraduate Dean and several current and past Deans have come from a GP background. The transition to focusing more on the secondary care side of the Deanery role should, however, not be underestimated.

Deputy Dean

Well, this does what it says on the tin. The Deputy deputises for the Dean at any and all meetings that the Dean cannot make. Usually the Deputy will have direct charge of aspects of the organisation and will lead on these on behalf of the Deanery. This may be recruitment of trainees, overseeing the HoSSs, in charge of all internal staff issues or leading on new initiatives within the Deanery (eg leadership programmes, bedside technology). The Deputy needs to work closely with the Dean and they need to share the same vision and strategic aims for the organisation. This role can expand greatly if the Dean gets involved in meetings at a UK-wide level (eg GMC committees). The Deputy is also able to undertake the appeals panels for the ARCP process. Meeting with

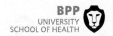

staff, dealing with work-based issues, understanding the training issues of the LEPs and being readily available and contactable for early intervention are also part of the role. Many new initiatives have come from those in the Deputy role which is a reflection not only on the skills they bring but also on the decentralised leadership style that the Dean may employ to maximise the input that said individuals bring to the table.

Postgraduate Dean

The Dean is in overall charge of the running and organisation of the Deanery. The lines of accountability for the Dean will vary depending on which UK country they are based. In Wales the Dean is responsible directly to the Welsh Government and in Scotland to the National Health Service Education Scotland. In Northern Ireland the Dean reports to the Chief Medical Officer and the Northern Ireland Assembly. In England they will be responsible to the LETB that they work in and then ultimately responsible to Health Education England.

Budgetary responsibility is a major task for any Dean particularly in times of financial constraint and proper financial governance is an essential element of the workings of any Deanery. The budget is typically negotiated on a year to year basis and can include the following:

- Trainee salaries
- Salaries of Deanery staff and extended staff (eg trainer grants)
- Non-staff costs such as libraries, postgraduate centres
- Removal expenses for trainees
- Provision of CPD for GPs
- Travel and subsistence for meeting attendance by all appropriate staff
- Costs of recruitment centres

These are just outline themes and many Deaneries have special projects that they fund which may be historical or in response to new initiatives to aid recruitment, bursaries, funding of higher degrees, conference attendance and presentation prizes and awards.

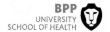

The overall number of staff on a Deanery payroll can stretch into hundreds when one considers the portfolio nature of the work many undertake in the community and hospital setting. Like any organisation this needs managing and ensuring that the environment is conducive to the recruitment and retention of the best staff.

The Dean is responsible for both the internal and external communication to ensure everyone understands the strategic direction of the organisation in a transparent and open way, including the overall breadth and depth of the work that the Deanery undertakes. As a Dean you will therefore find yourself chairing various conferences, meetings and producing publications to ensure this understanding is fully realised.

While the GMC as the regulator is responsible for setting standards and quality assuring the training, the Dean is responsible for the quality management of those standards. This will involve commissioning visits to every educational provider (Trusts, Health Boards and practices) in the area and ensuring that the quality standards are being met and that the Deanery is getting value for money for the educational investment it makes on behalf of its health department. The Dean is responsible for these visits and can use them to develop a better relationship with each educational provider. The role is not about policing the health organisations but about working together, openly, to resolve any outstanding quality of training issues and problems a Trust may face. However, if these problems are not resolvable then it is the responsibility of the Dean, in conjunction with the GMC, to move the trainees to a more appropriate educational environment. These are the most difficult decisions the Dean will have to make as invariably it will have an impact on the local provision of services. These decisions potentially get escalated into the political arena with the local politicians seeking to understand the decision-making process. It is therefore essential that the Dean has an open, transparent process that is fully understood by the LEPs and others.

Reporting to health officials, answering questions from politicians and Ministers and meeting with Chief Executives and Medical Directors of the local Health Boards/Trusts are all part of the job of a Dean.

For their own support Deans do attend the Conference of Postgraduate Medical and Dental Deans (COPMeD).

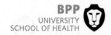

COPMeD is the Conference Of Postgraduate Medical Deans (UK). It provides a focus for those responsible for the strategic overview and operational delivery of postgraduate medical training in the four nations of the United Kingdom, and by ensuring excellent training, is a key player in maintaining quality of care and patient safety.

(COPMeD website as of 10 May 2017)

COPMeD meets for a residential meeting about three times a year. It is an excellent networking opportunity and provides peer support to the Deans. It is an opportunity for any updates from the GMC, the Academy of Royal Colleges and Medical Schools Council to present any new initiatives that have a UK-wide impact. It allows for updates from the four nations and updates on the Gold Guide, which outlines the rules surrounding the employment and processes of training. It also enables the British Medical Association junior doctor representatives to discuss any issues they may have related to training and the consistency of approach to training across the UK.

The majority of Deans do work full time in the role but a few have still chosen to keep a hand in their chosen specialty; of those most do no more than two sessions per week.

Chapter summary

Careers in postgraduate medical education typically link with Postgraduate Deaneries and LETBs across all of the UK. Roles range from the ES through to TPD, HoSS and then on to wider cross-specialty portfolios. As you progress the greater the level of influence you will be likely to have.

Key points

- Look at your local Deanery website to see the breadth of positions available.

- Talk to those currently in post.

- Be vocal about your desire to work in education.

- Think about getting a higher certification in medical education.

- Do not forget about an MBA.

- See if there are bursaries or grants to help with the costs.

- Let your partners/department/family know of your intentions.

- Enthusiasm and interest are key attributes.

Useful resources

Committee of General Practice Education Directors (CoGPED) – www.cogped.org.uk

Conference of Postgraduate Medical Deans (COPMeD) – www.copmed.org.uk

General Medical Council (2017) *Generic Professional Capabilities Framework*. [Online]. Available at: www.gmc-uk.org/education/postgraduate/GPC.asp [Accessed 21 June 2017].

The Gold Guide (2016) 6th edition. [Online]. Available at: www.copmed.org.uk [Accessed 21 June 2017].

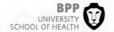

Chapter 4

Chapter 5

NHS, government and Royal College medical education roles

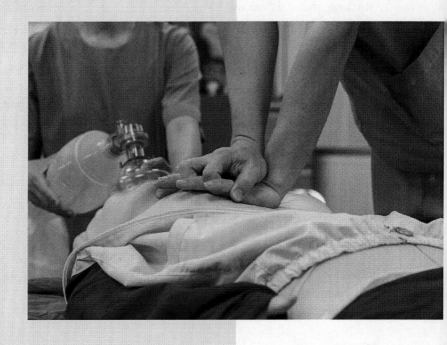

Introduction

In this chapter, we will describe career pathways in NHS, government and Royal College (RC) settings. As with all these areas there is significant overlap in terms of a portfolio or potential portfolio career for you. So, if you were in a senior NHS education role you will interact with RCs, government, undergraduate (UG) or postgraduate (PG) organisations depending on the issues at hand.

National Health Service (NHS) roles

The NHS exists to deliver high-quality care to all. Aneurin Bevan authored the NHS Act 1946 that became live on 5 July 1948 in England and Wales establishing a national health service free at the point of need and paid for by public monies.

So although medicine in its broadest terms has developed and innovated beyond all recognition in the last 50 years, with advances for example in technology, a key requirement remains: the training of staff. Without highly trained and up to date staff there is no NHS.

As with all medical education roles, you will usually dabble with a number of them and there is no single pathway. A common starting point is taking on an educational role in your specialty in the employing NHS organisation. This initial step into an educational role is typically driven by your own clinical expertise and/or interests.

Working in an education role in a Health Board or Trust in the UK will frequently overlap with those in UG and PG. The General Medical Council (GMC) refers to NHS bodies as the Local Education Providers (LEPs) and the standards that apply to UG and PG apply similarly to LEPs.

So, your employer is likely to be the NHS and most organisations will or should have an education and training strategy to help guide developments.

Most NHS healthcare providers in the UK will have set out a vision and values that they adhere to. Dorset HealthCare University NHS Foundation Trust as one example states its values as follows (as of 10 May 2017):

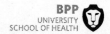

Working together for patients
Respect and dignity
Commitment to quality care
Compassion
Improving lives
Everyone counts
Commitment to learning

A global example is the Princeton Health System (its website as of 10 May 2017):

Vision Statement of Princeton HealthCare System

Princeton HealthCare System is a premier, integrated healthcare system that strives to anticipate and respond to the lifelong needs of the residents of Central New Jersey and beyond by providing excellent clinical care. Princeton HealthCare System is recognized for its commitment to enhancing the health of its community; providing superior services to its patients, delivering outstanding value, embracing clinical innovations; providing exceptional medical and health education; and supporting a knowledgeable, skilled and caring medical and employee staff.

The Mission of Princeton HealthCare System is to be the focal point of a comprehensive community health system that responds to the healthcare needs of our service area residents. Princeton HealthCare System will provide inpatient and outpatient care, community health education, medical education, and should promote medical and scientific research when appropriate. It is integral to the Mission of Princeton HealthCare System to continually improve quality of service to our patients and community and to provide appropriate healthcare to all.

As we describe in Chapter 2, frequently you will start your medical education career with a broad portfolio dabbling in UG, PG, and perhaps college roles. This broad portfolio is very useful in providing you with a range of experience and enables you to develop skills and networks and enhance your reputation as a doctor who prioritises education and training. Reputations in medical education are as important as they are in the clinical setting.

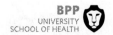

Case study

My journey in medical education started out in my own specialty. I was the first consultant in Liaison Psychiatry appointed in my Trust. It became apparent really quickly that my colleagues in A&E and on the acute medical wards did not understand my role and the new service was met with a mixed reception.

I spoke to the Clinical Director of A&E and explained that if all the staff in the department used the liaison service appropriately we could triage patients better.

I then set up a monthly programme of what I called awareness training for all A&E staff, timing the sessions to cover all different shifts and all professions. Over a period of three or four months all staff attended. After this there was a real change in the nature and type of referrals and I was able to skill up a number of the A&E staff to take on initial assessments of risk of certain patients. This experience was borne out of necessity but really showed me the impact that a targeted training could have on patient care.

Case study

I had always been involved in bedside teaching for all staff. I noticed that one of the common themes was the lack of confidence that junior doctors and nurses had in interpreting ECGs. It struck me that we needed an ongoing training programme for all staff on this. With two colleagues I devised a two-hour training session open to all staff with an open tutorial session once a month where anyone could bring not just ECG questions but also questions or issues about any aspect of the care on the Coronary Care Unit and on the medical wards.

The keenest to learn were the nurses who frankly had more hours' contact with the patients and who in many ways were best placed to undertake this. These sessions still run today eight years after we set them up. I published not a study but a description of the learning and as a result I was approached by the Trust to roll out similar sessions to all staff.

BPP
UNIVERSITY
SCHOOL OF HEALTH

So, you may start with a full-time NHS contract with Direct Clinical Care and Supporting Professional Activity sessions all linked to clinical work then gradually add in sessions for UG or PG medical education roles with dedicated time.

Drivers for any NHS Trust/Health Board are quality of service to patients and financial balancing of the books. In terms of medical education as an LEP the organisation will be directly accountable to the GMC for the standards. Some direct quotes from the standards relevant to LEPs include:

Organisations must make sure that learners have an appropriate level of clinical supervision at all times by an experienced and competent supervisor, who can advise or attend as needed. The level of supervision must fit the individual learner's competence, confidence and experience. The support and clinical supervision must be clearly outlined to the learner and the supervisor.

Organisations must design rotas to:

(a) Make sure doctors in training have appropriate clinical supervision

(b) Support doctors in training to develop the professional values, knowledge, skills and behaviours required of all doctors working in the UK

(c) Provide learning opportunities that allow doctors in training to meet the requirements of their curriculum and training programme

(d) Give doctors in training access to educational supervisors

(e) Minimise the adverse effects of fatigue and workload

Doctors in training must have protected time for learning while they are doing clinical or medical work, or during academic training, and for attending organised educational sessions, training days, courses and other learning opportunities to meet the requirements of their curriculum. In timetabled educational sessions, doctors in training must not be interrupted for service unless there is an exceptional and unanticipated clinical need to maintain patient safety.

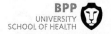
BPP
UNIVERSITY
SCHOOL OF HEALTH

> LEPs control the organisational culture and the quality of education and training in their local organisations. An executive must be accountable for educational governance, and those in educational leadership roles must have demonstrable educational credibility and capability.
>
> Organisations responsible for managing and providing education and training must monitor how educational resources are allocated and used, including ensuring time in trainers' job plans.

These will give you a feel for the drivers that you will face and the opportunities mapped to the GMC standards that you can influence and hence make a significant and lasting difference in the Health Board or Trust.

NHS medical education career pathway

The significant overlap between all of these education roles is underpinned by the final common denominator: high-quality training and education equates with better services and care to patients. In an NHS organisation or any healthcare provider a medical education role is frequently combined with responsibility for training a range of professionals and not necessarily restricted to just medical students, trainees, consultants, General Practitioners (GPs) or Staff and Associate Specialists (SASs). This diversity may suit your own needs and interests and is something to consider when planning a medical educator role (see Chapter 2).

In terms of the career progression Table 5.1 shows some examples of lead roles in education within NHS organisations:

Training and education roles in the NHS
Audit lead
Service innovation lead
Quality improvement lead
Resuscitation training
Major incident training/rehearsal
Revalidation lead

Table 5.1 Training and education roles in the NHS

So, you may start by leading within your specialty and then move on to looking at an educational role for your hospital and then typically an Associate Medical Director (AMD) for Education. These roles are also termed Directors of Medical Education and may include responsibility for trainees, medical student placements and post Certificate of Completion of Training (CCT) continuing professional development (CPD) in the organisation. These roles do differ across the UK and some will also include medical workforce planning or governance.

Your interfaces will be with Health Boards/Trust Boards, local PG Deanery/Local Education and Training Boards (LETB) and medical schools, RCs and healthcare service regulators such as the Care Quality Commission in England and Health Inspectorate Wales. There is such an overlap between quality of training and quality of service to patients. In a department with poor outcomes for patients there is highly likely to be sub-standard training and learning experiences.

Usually a Health Board or Trust will appoint a range of AMD posts to support the Medical Director (MD). These can include a range of areas of responsibility, including research, workforce, quality assurance, governance and/or revalidation to name but a few. Therefore, you will be part of a team of AMDs. This position gives you real opportunities to learn about others' roles. From the AMD role there are options to move into a medical leadership role such as MD or to continue a path in medical education into UG, PG or RCs. All of these roles should be seen as stepping-stones to other portfolios.

Case study

I had been a GP for five years or so and had started to have registrars on placement with me in practice. Through conversations with the trainees it was obvious that quite a few of them were apprehensive about being a partner. They didn't feel confident enough. I had been involved in the local medical school helping to deliver communications teaching to second and third years and also had helped to set up a peer to peer mentoring scheme for students. It struck me that the GP registrars might benefit from this as well. I discussed this with a few colleagues, surveyed the trainees at the next regional

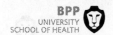

training day and there was clearly an appetite not just for a peer mentoring but also for a mentoring scheme per se.

We used a local hospital PG centre to deliver the first session for potential mentors and this triggered interest in the hospital. This led to a regional mentoring scheme for any doctor in any specialty. This work really showed me the impact that a simple idea can have and spurred me on to eventually seek out the AMD role the next year.

Case study

A morning in the life of an Associate Medical Director (Director of Medical Education)

8:30am. I have to chair an interview to appoint a lead clinician for resuscitation within the Trust. This had been an unfilled post for approximately 12 months. It was really affecting the organisation's ability to have a co-ordinated approach to resuscitation training across not just all specialties in medicine but the whole organisation for all staff. There had been a number of major issues with the Health Board not wanting to release funding. I spent some time, in essence, arguing/discussing with individual members of the Trust Board that without this clinical lead which could be a medic or a non-medic that patient safety was compromised. In the end there was an agreement that whoever was appointed to this role would require one day a week and then the payment would follow, ie if it was a medic, they would be paid at consultant level and as a non-medic they would be paid at an appropriate level. As it was there were only two candidates, both of whom were doctors. I chaired the interview panel and we had a number of representatives from across different professional and clinical areas. This was quite an easy decision as clearly one of the consultants had significant experience in resuscitation training and had a UK role in the area. So in the end all the meetings I attended to find the funding for this role was time well spent.

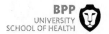

10:30am. I went straight from the interviews to a CPD session that was part of an ongoing programme that I had set up for all consultants and SAS doctors. This two-hour session was in regard to the requirements of appraisal and revalidation and I had asked a Responsible Officer from a neighbouring Trust to come in and discuss their experience of the key issues with the consultants and SAS doctors. So my role in that session was essentially to act as chair and lead discussions. The session was very interactive and the feedback from the attendees was very positive.

12:30pm. I stopped for half an hour for a sandwich and to check on some emails and to make a couple of phone calls. One in particular was to the AMD for Quality, thinking of a meeting that we had later on in the week.

1:00–1:30pm. I met with the administrator secretary who worked half time supporting my role. The purpose of the meeting was to start pulling together the paperwork in what we considered to be the potential response to a GMC visit to the region in about six months' time. We focused on the red flags in the GMC survey that we had and specifically focusing on those red flags over two or more years in a particular department. I tasked her with looking at these at-risk areas and the departments and planned to meet again in two weeks' time in order to devise the battle plan.

1:30–2:00pm. I had been invited to a meeting with the local medical school in regards to the issue of dedicated time for consultants and SAS doctors to teach the medical students. This was just one more meeting in a series of meetings I had about this issue. With job planning we had come to a deal for the bulk of consultants and SAS doctors who were teaching. But there were still some doctors whose job plans were so complex that we weren't able to come to an agreement. This remained a frustration for me.

In the NHS most MDs have executive responsibility for medical education at board level in their organisation. This will usually mean leading a team of AMDs and working very closely with other directors such as Nursing, Operations Director and development as well as the Chief Executive Officer (CEO).

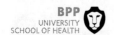

Case study

I have been an MD for four years now and key to me getting to this point in my career has been people who have supported me, and who I have learnt from. If there is one single experience that helped the most in preparing me for this role it was the three years I was an AMD. In that role I had responsibility for education and workforce planning as the two go together. What helped me the most was covering for the MD when she was on leave. Up until that point, I really hadn't appreciated the level of responsibility and the wide range of 'problems' that landed on the MD's desk. These ranged from complex disciplinary issues to rota gaps. Also of real use was working very closely with the CEO and Director of Finance. Also I saw for the first time the impact of politics on decision-making. I had not appreciated that and I learnt a lot from both of them.

So, in the NHS there are great opportunities to teach directly day to day within the job and to expand your training and education role into formal roles and responsibilities. Within the NHS there are possibly more opportunities to get involved in interprofessional and multidisciplinary education and training due to the nature of the environment (Barr, 2002).

Government medical education roles

In the UK all health matters are now devolved from Westminster to the administrations in England, Scotland, Northern Ireland and Wales. In each of the four nations health matters including medical education have developed differently. Each have their own processes for managing policy for medical education and each have different processes for commissioning and managing UG and PG medical education. There has been, in recent years, a divergence of the underpinning principles in the NHS in the different countries. Despite these differences, there is a global UK dimension in regard to medical education and irrespective of which country you are working in there will be similar issues albeit with local nuances.

If the role of Government is to set the policy for the NHS then there is clearly a significant overlap between service delivery on

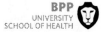

the one hand and training and education on the other. In order to meet the projected workforce demands of a particular service model once a Government sets a policy for, say, the profile of the specialties in the UK Foundation Programme, this will have a knock-on effect on medical schools, and then specialty training and service delivery. All are interlinked.

Government Departments of Health are by their nature complex but all UK countries will have a Minister for Health or equivalent role. The Department of Health (DH) England on its website (as of 10 May 2017) states:

What we do

The Department of Health (DH) helps people to live better for longer. We lead, shape and fund health and care in England, making sure people have the support, care and treatment they need, with the compassion, respect and dignity they deserve.

DH is a ministerial department, supported by 29 agencies and public bodies.

And so for medical education careers within DH England a member of the senior team includes the Chief Medical Officer (CMO) for England. In addition, one of the public bodies supporting DH is Health Education England (HEE). This organisational structure highlights the link between Government and UG and PG medical education.

HEE, originally set up as a Special Health Authority in 2012, has been a non-departmental public body since April 2015. On HEE's website (as of 10 May 2017):

HEE exists for one reason only: to support the delivery of excellent healthcare and health improvement to the patients and public of England by ensuring that the workforce of today and tomorrow has the right numbers, skills, values and behaviours, at the right time and in the right place.

Also for example, in Scotland on the government website (as of 10 May 2017) it states:

The Scottish Government Health and Social Care Directorate aims to help people sustain and improve their health, especially in disadvantaged communities, ensuring better, local and faster access to healthcare.

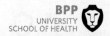

> *The Directorate also allocates resources and sets the strategic direction for NHS Scotland and is responsible for the development and implementation of health and social care policy.*

NHS Education for Scotland (NES) is responsible for medical training and education. On the NES website (as of 10 May 2017) it states:

> *Our vision is to provide quality education for a healthy Scotland*

> *Our mission is to provide education that enables excellence in health and care for the people of Scotland*

> *NES is an education and training body and a special health board within NHS Scotland, with responsibility of developing and delivering education and training for the healthcare workforce in Scotland*

Opportunities to get involved at government level can fall into a range of options. All UK nations have a CMO whose role is to advise respective governments on all aspects of 'medicine'. Most CMOs have come from a public health background as a lot of policy rightly focuses on that area. CMOs are the professional lead for all doctors in the relevant country.

Policy development will require you to have an in-depth understanding of your area, the service, training and education issues and any other consequences. Within these roles there is a lot of stakeholder engagement, data gathering, sense checking and the drafting and redrafting of the policy paper.

Looking at the annual CMO report can be very useful for you to get a sense of what is politically 'hot' and give you a understanding of the policy stance and ethos of the respective health departments.

The four Governments do have different policies and depending where you will work the focus will invariably be different. So as one example in Wales a new policy for organ donation was put in place with presumed opt-in. For this policy to be implemented it would have taken many people working in a team at civil servant, national adviser and CMO level.

Supporting each CMO will usually be a Deputy, civil servants in the respective DH and Senior Medical Advisers/Officers with specific portfolios or national leads in specific areas or service themes. So for example one role could be national lead for primary care responsible for advising the Health Minister on the delivery

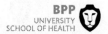

of service and advising Ministers on policy. Invariably this also means influencing national policy on education, UG and PG and post-CCT in primary care in this example.

So reflecting on the career pathway it is common for you to have had experience at UG, PG or college level in that particular field and then moved into an advisory role or national lead in Government.

Case study

I had been a consultant in community paediatrics for 12 years or so and had also been Regional Adviser for the college. I had sat on a number of college committees looking at policy and service standards for community services. I also had a particular interest in disability rights and had a further portfolio working in the local PG Deanery as an Associate Dean. In one particular national group I was working very closely with the then Deputy CMO who inspired me to consider a role in Government. Talking to her revealed areas that I was unaware of, namely that Health Ministers need accurate advice from the shop floor in order to make policy decisions. I shadowed the DCMO for a few days and this really opened my eyes. About a year later a job was advertised as an adviser for child services and the DCMO supported and encouraged me to apply. A key difference for me was that I was going to have to cease all clinical practice as the government role was a full-time job. I did apply and was successful. The role is demanding and challenging. I am just one of a wide team of advisers and one challenge is to ensure we join up our thinking. The rewards are great in that I can see policy decisions being actioned and patients and their families benefiting. I have learnt that once the Minister makes a public statement that something will happen, it happens. It can feel like a slow process but we get there.

On a day to day basis as an adviser, for example you could and will get called at very short notice to advise the Minister on a subject that a member of public has just raised or an opposition Member of Parliament has asked about. You will need to be on your toes, preparing replies for the Minister, briefings, speeches and letters.

There are somewhat different skills required at this level. Policy drafting cannot be undertaken in isolation so a lot of the work is visiting hospitals and community facilities and talking with staff, patients, local council representatives and the voluntary sector so that you are in a position to advise and brief when needed.

Case study
A day in the life of a Deputy Chief Medical Officer

8:00am. I had a pre-meeting with civil servant colleagues to brief me on the latest recruitment figures into GP training posts and the current status of GP partners who had retired and the vacancies at that level. This was in preparation for a meeting I was having at 9am with the PG Dean and her team.

9:00am. In the meeting my aim was to get a clear view for the Minister about the scope of the current gaps, impact on patient care and what we could do as a government. A key issue discussed at length was the need for us to be innovative in regard to the use of a wider non-medical workforce.

10:15am. I met again with civil servant colleagues and two of the policy advisers for GP joined us and we discussed the option for the Minister to announce a set of measures to help reverse the trends.

11:00am. This was a meeting with a Head of a local medical school who wanted to discuss government funding of bursaries for Physician Associates. We agreed that this was in principle a very good idea and he was going to send me details and a paper that I could turn into a ministerial briefing to help get the money confirmed.

12:00pm. I had a routine longstanding regular visit to a local A&E department where I made a point of spending time with the staff, having a cup of coffee and getting their views on how things could be improved.

3:00pm. Back in the office and as I arrived, one of my public health colleagues was there with recent data on measles numbers. We were very close to a significant outbreak and we agreed that he should liaise with the media team to organise a piece for the BBC and ITV.

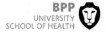

3:30pm. I had 30 minutes, which I used to read through a document about renal dialysis services across the region. There had been concerns about the capacity of the service and a case had been put to Government for additional funding to extend a wing. I needed to understand the issues in some detail so I would be in a position to brief the CMO.

4:00pm. I had my regular weekly meeting with the Health Minister with myself, the CMO and a few national leads.

6:00pm. Finish.

There is so much overlap and interdependency between all these medical education roles. So for example, as a Head of Medical School you will be employed by a university and, even though the university is an independent institution, the respective Government will set the policy for medical schools, you interface with other medical schools, the UK Foundation Programme Office and your local PG Deanery/LETBs. In terms of PG medical education the four Governments have different infrastructures, processes and systems. In Northern Ireland the PG Deanery sits within the devolved Government; in Scotland the PG Deanery sits with NES which overarches all health commissioning and then advises the Government.

Royal College (RC) medical education careers

All Royal Colleges in the UK are professional membership organisations and are registered charities. The purpose of colleges in general is to improve patient care and to support their members. As an example the Royal College of Surgeons (RCS) England on its home page states (as of 10 May 2017):

Mission statement

The RCS of England is committed to enabling surgeons to achieve and maintain the highest standards of surgical practice and patient care.

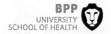

In terms of education/training what the college statement says it does is:

Supervise training of surgeons in approved posts

Provide educational and practical workshops for surgeons and other medical professionals at all stages of their careers

Examine trainees to ensure the highest professional standards

Provide support and advice for surgeons in all stages of their career

Act as an advisory body to the department of health, health authorities, trusts, hospitals and other professional bodies

There are a number of routes into a medical education career in an RC. As a newly appointed or relatively newly appointed consultant or GP, the college examinations are still fresh in your mind and you might get involved as a college examiner. After some experience of this role you may then move on to perhaps representing a region on the college examination board. Then, if you have the skills and enthusiasm, an option is to move on to chair that board (see Chapter 6).

Typically each college will have regional divisions or equivalent and that is an excellent platform for you to enhance your career. So if your college has a division in your region, there will be opportunities for leading on a range of portfolios such as careers, research and clinical-based portfolios.

Examples of Royal College/Faculty roles
College Tutor
Regional Advisers
Educators/trainer recognition
Audit/Quality improvement
Continuing professional development
Examinations
Professional standards
Professional affairs

Examples of Royal College/Faculty roles
Quality management
Curriculum development
Regional ambassadors
Specialised eg e-learning

Table 5.2 Examples of Royal College/Faculty roles

A key college role is the College Tutor (CT). Different colleges have different selection processes for recruitment into CT roles and the job descriptions are diverse. The common theme is that the CT acts as an organiser and co-ordinator of training for trainees in that specialty and is the voice of the college at a local level and a key link between the Trust/Health Board, local PG Deanery/LETB and the college. In a CT role there is a need for close working with your local Deanery/LETB representatives. Therefore, good networking and communication skills are required.

All colleges have college assessors whose role it is to represent the relevant college at Advisory Appointments Committees. These are legally constituted interview panels set up by the appointing NHS employer and have to have a college assessor. This is a key role with the remit of advising the employer on the suitability or otherwise of each candidate. The purpose is to maintain standards of practice and enabling a consistent and reliable assessment of the training of individual candidates.

All colleges will have a Regional Advisor (RA) who co-ordinates and supports the network of CTs. In addition, the RA reviews all the job descriptions and person specifications prior to any consultant post going out to advert. Some RAs are also Heads of Specialty School for their region. This latter role is a PG Deanery role (see Chapter 4) but again there is considerable overlap.

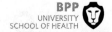

Case study

I had been a CT in Anaesthesia in my local hospital. There were three of us across the Trust covering the three sites. I did this role for a number of years and sat on the local Specialist Training Committee (STC). I had a number of excellent role models on the STC and one in particular encouraged me to get more involved across the region. One thing I did was set up a peer group for all the CTs across the region as it was clear from feedback that some in the smaller units felt quite isolated. I then became Deputy RA and then RA. In my role I manage and support the network of CTs and I have to say that the fact I had been a tutor for five years does give me a good understanding of the difficulties faced in the role. I work very closely with the Subdean for Quality and Governance in the local PG Deanery. We have a shared agenda, which is high-quality training that meets the GMC standards. In my RA role I was also able to get involved at a national level in the design of the assessment elements of the curriculum for anaesthesia due to my interest in simulation learning.

Case study

I had dabbled with e-learning back in the day when it was in its infancy. I could see that there were a lot of resources that could be accessed online and that for example any training I delivered in ENT surgery I put pictures and text on the web for the trainees to pre-read. To encourage the trainees to publish we had a number of presentations accepted at the college national conferences one year. There was quite a lot of interest and I was contacted a few months later and asked if I would sit on the college online learning group. This evolved into the e-portfolio group and because of my interest I was asked to chair this. Because of the work the college published and working links with DH I was invited to be a member of a DH group looking at e-learning for all healthcare in the region.

Career opportunities may and will arise because of developments in technology-enhanced learning and in innovative workforce developments such as the Physicians Associates (PAs). Extracts from the Royal College of Physicians (RCP) website (as of 10 May 2017) state for example:

> *The Education department at the Royal College of Physicians takes a leading role in developing educational policy and initiatives and in providing a number of services and resources to support the professional development of doctors. A range of high quality educational programmes are designed and delivered by the Education team in addition to developing elearning modules and delivering valued revalidation and CPD resources.*

> *Vice-President for Education and Training (VPET) The VPET is a senior college officer, reporting directly to the President of the RCP, a professional membership organisation. The VPET works closely with the Director of Education and Head of Revalidation and CPD to deliver strategic objectives and develop new opportunities.*

So with this just as an example, within the RCP there is a new Faculty of PA established within the college whose role is to represent and provide professional support to PAs across the UK. From the RCP site (as of 10 May 2017):

> *Members of the faculty will be part of a professional membership body that will campaign for progress and change in the profession, advise government, and take part in national debates on medical, clinical and public health issues.*

All RCs have a set of standards for clinical service and most will provide NHS organisations with formal reviews of clinical service. These 'invited reviews' are usually undertaken by a visiting team and this is another excellent career opportunity for you to get involved with. Although these reviews are invited by the NHS organisations to review the quality of service, there is such an overlap that training and education issues are frequently commented on. Also the processes and skills required/learnt through participating in these processes can stand you in good stead.

In the UK the RCs devise and write the relevant specialty curricula which then go through an approval process in the GMC. Hence all colleges will need individuals who have experience of curriculum design.

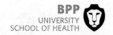

All colleges have a committee structure so if you are not sure look up their website and more importantly network. Talk to people. As we have said, medical education is about people.

Case study

My career pathway in medical education was fairly typical. I had been a CT for a number of years and then a TPD for surgery. At the same time I was a college examiner and had been part of a subgroup that revised the professional standards. The Head of Specialty School in the region retired and I was successful, encouraged by my colleagues. This afforded me the chance with both College and Deanery Head of Specialty School roles to make significant changes to how we delivered training. The Head of Specialty School was a high profile role, in the press and media. In this role I learnt a lot, interacting with government civil servants. Then the role of professional affairs for the college was developed and I was encouraged by colleagues in both the college and my own clinical department to apply and was successful. This role was very challenging, as I hadn't really appreciated the political dimension to the work. I worked very closely with all the key organisations: HEE, DH, the Medical Schools Council and the GMC.

A formal medical education role in the NHS, government and/or RC invariably overlap and complement each other and can be a stepping-stone to more influential roles.

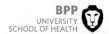

Chapter summary

In NHS medical education roles there are a range of specialty-specific and then more generic roles. Government roles in medical education can be extremely varied and you will advise Ministers and help devise policy. In RC roles there are again a wide array of interesting roles, from delivering and designing CPD to examining and leading curriculum development.

Key points

- There are a range of opportunities to influence at different levels.

- Whichever career pathway you choose there are links between them all.

- You can start your medical education portfolio career in any area and use the experience and skills acquired as a stepping-stone on to other areas.

Useful resources

General Medical Council (2015) *Promoting excellence: standards for medical education and training*. [Online]. Available at: www.gmc-uk.org/education/standards.asp [Accessed 21 June 2017].

Princeton HealthCare System – www.princetonhcs.org/phcs-home/what-we-stand-for/vision-statement.aspx

References

Barr, H (2002) *Inter-professional Education: Today, Yesterday and Tomorrow*: *A review*. London: Learning and Teaching Support Network, Centre for Health Sciences and Practice.

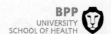

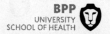

Chapter 6

Prepare – which qualifications, why, when and where?

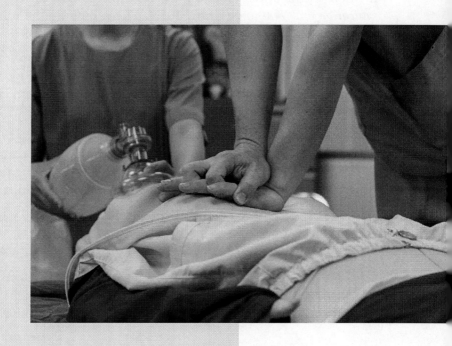

Introduction

Why do you need to objectively demonstrate your competency as a medical educator?

Relicensing, revalidation and job plans have shone a spotlight on the composition of the working week. Every aspect of the job plan must be justified and you must demonstrate that you have the skills and qualifications to undertake the roles you have chosen. It is relatively simple to demonstrate your clinical qualifications via membership of your professional college and your updated record of your continuing professional development (CPD) and yearly appraisal. The question is: what evidence can you present mapped to your role as an educator? How do you know your job plan for the education time will be agreed or even understood?

The key to the future is the professionalisation of the role of educators and following on from that is the requirement to have recognised qualifications and ability for the role. What does this mean in a practical sense from the start of your career in education on to whatever future pathway you choose?

The General Medical Council (GMC) has now defined the standards in their publication *Promoting Excellence: Standards for Medical Education and Training* (GMC, 2015). These include the following five themes:

1. Learning environment and culture. This is about the environment being safe for patients and supportive for learners and teachers. It includes the role of the organisation in fostering the educational agenda.

2. Educational governance and leadership. This is designed to continuously improve the quality outcomes of education and training. This is done by measuring performance against the standards, demonstrating accountability and responding when standards are not being met.

3. Supporting learners. This involves the support that learners can expect both in educational and pastoral terms to achieve the curriculum requirements.

4. Supporting educators. This is the main standard that is directly applicable to any and every doctor involved in education or

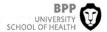

supervision. It is really the starting point or foundation on which to build your educational career. The GMC is clear now that the educators should be selected, inducted, trained and appraised to reflect their education and training responsibilities. This is a very new standard to which the GMC will hold the Local Education Providers accountable to deliver. These standards from the regulator provide you with the leverage within the appraisal and job planning process to set out your educational needs explicitly and highlight the time you need to perform the educator role.

5. Developing and implementing curricula and assessments. This theme is about being able to ensure that the medical schools achieve the learning outcomes required for graduates and in the postgraduate arena, the curricula and assessments are implemented so trainees can demonstrate what is expected and can show they have achieved the learning outcomes required by their curriculum.

These themes and associated standards represent the start of the requirements within the workplace and also the start of the journey. Taking on additional roles in medical education will involve you in enhancing your knowledge and skills to deliver your professional role. It really is your choice to pick the course or courses that will help your own development and indeed promotion.

The range of courses is vast, from local half-day skills workshops, online learning to Certificates, Diplomas, Master's and PhDs. Clearly some of these options will just incur your time rather than require you to pay. Indeed many education organisations provide courses free of charge to ensure the maximum number of educational and clinical supervisors comply with the new GMC educator and clinical supervisor regulations.

There are a number of questions for you to answer for yourself.

1. **What are your developmental needs?**

   The advent of revalidation has introduced reflective practice and the need to undertake 360 degree questionnaires and these may help enormously in focusing both on your current skills and also unmet needs in medical education. These reflections can be used as a springboard for your further development and job planning process. Cast your net widely in finding who can

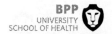

best advise you on both your aptitude and skills in delivering teaching and training. The 360 degree questions should certainly have a section related to your current educational role and this evidence can be used positively within the appraisal process.

2. **What educational career aspirations do you have?**

Many of you will know the expense of revision courses for college examinations. This is clearly an investment in your clinical future. It is no different when investing in your medical education career. Higher qualifications will need money, time and the commitment principally of yourself but also potentially your departmental colleagues and employer.

Despite your enthusiasm for the subject there will be many competing pressures on your time and you do need to be realistic about the commitment you are going to make. Clinical work, family, friends and a work–life balance are important. They, of course, are the same pressures that you will already have encountered and should not diminish your drive in medical education.

3. **When?**

Again, it is worth re-emphasising exactly what your career aspirations in medical education will be. Substantive roles in medical education will require at least some form of university-recognised certification, if only to demonstrate your commitment to the subject on your Curriculum Vitae. Undertaking a university-accredited Certificate, Diploma, Master's or PhD in Medical Education will need a substantial time commitment above and beyond your day job. You need to consider the level of support you can expect to get, not just at work but also at home. Will your employer fund the course? Will the Deanery give you a bursary? Will you get any protected time in the week to undertake the reading and assessments required?

That having been said, more and more doctors are undertaking these additional qualifications at an earlier stage of their career. There are now intercalated bachelor's degrees in medical education being offered in some medical schools. Many academic foundation programmes include medical education as an option and many lead to a Certificate in Medical Education. So perhaps the earlier you start, the more options may present to you over your career. Some however choose to only acquire higher certification after achieving the Royal College exams in their specialty. This is an individual choice and for some is a sensible approach to ensure that the clinical aspects of your career are progressing smoothly and you focus on the curriculum requirements of your chosen specialty.

Case study

I have always been interested in teaching. My primary degree before going into medical school was in chemistry and I worked for a few years as a freelance tutor and really enjoyed it. One of the reasons I chose this medical school was that it had an intercalated BSc in medical education. The course was very intensive but well worth the effort and time. I was hesitant about dropping out of my year for the 12 months but feel this qualification and the level of understanding and skills I now have will help me in my career.

4. **Where to study?**

A simple online search for medical education courses produces hundreds of hits not just in the UK but around the globe. There is therefore no lack of opportunities to enrol on courses. The key is to personalise exactly what it is you want from your studies and what will be of use to your career. Advice is easy to find as many of your colleagues will be happy to share their experiences and advise on the best possible courses. Practical issues always need to be considered. How local is the course? How long does it run for? Does it demand your attendance personally or is it a distance learning course you can do in your own time? How much are the fees?

Different levels of learning

There are of course different levels of learning, from half-day tasters to one-week workshops through to formal university-accredited qualifications from Certificate up to PhD. We will discuss options for your learning in two main themes, CPD and formal qualifications.

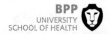

Continuing Professional Development (CPD)

A good starting point is the Academy of Medical Educators *Professional Standards for Medical, Dental and Veterinary Educators* (AoME, 2014). These standards describe a range of practice domains underpinned by core values. The domains are described in Table 6.1.

Academy of Medical Educators (AoME) practice domains
1.   Designing and planning learning
2.   Teaching and facilitating learning
3.   Assessment of learning
4.   Educational research and scholarship
5.   Educational management and leadership

Table 6.1 Academy of Medical Educators (AoME) practice domains

These domains and the descriptors within each are a good starting point for you to consider your learning needs. There are other important areas that you should seek out, including learning in change management and media training.

Change management

In any medical education role you will be involved in or in fact lead on significant change within your organisation. Change management is a complex process and requires a specific skill set. There are a range of courses that can help you to acquire these skills and one as an example is PRINCE2 (an acronym for **PR**ojects **IN** Controlled Environments). This is a process-based method that is widely used internationally. There are different levels, most starting with PRINCE2 Foundation which covers the basics and then at a higher level the PRINCE2 Practitioner.

Change management links with quality improvement and having an understanding of basic processes such as the **Plan** … **Do** … **Study** … **Act** (PDSA) cycle. The PDSA model is attributed to Edward Deming (1983) and is frequently used to manage continuous improvement in both clinical and educational environments.

BPP
UNIVERSITY
SCHOOL OF HEALTH

Media training

Dealing with the media has become an increasing part of the role in response to issues that crop up. In the postgraduate arena this could include media scrutiny on any ongoing difficulties of recruiting to certain specialties. Also, there may be patches in the locality that are particularly hard to fill and the lack of recruitment has a knock-on effect to service delivery within the hospital part of the rotations. In an undergraduate setting the impact of the selection criteria and pass rates may be under scrutiny. The media will seek statements and interviews from a 'spokesperson' from the relevant organisation. You may also be asked to answer questions from Members of Parliament or Ministers with regard to learning or training in your organisation. These questions can have a fast turnaround time so it is essential that you are aware of who you can turn to in your organisation who can source accurate data to allow for a timely reply.

Formal qualifications

There are a range of providers in the UK including:

1. University taught programmes
2. University internal programmes
3. Royal Colleges

1. University taught programmes

In the UK the following universities all run Master's degrees in medical education, most of which can be done by distance learning rather than face to face which can be difficult to organise around work commitments.

- University of Liverpool
- University of East Anglia
- University of Warwick
- University of Manchester
- University of Dundee
- University of Cardiff
- University of Keele
- University of Edinburgh
- University of Nottingham

While the above list is not exhaustive, it does show a wide coverage of the UK and the prominence of the degree. Do

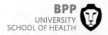

remember that even if you choose not to undertake a local course the advent of distance learning packages allows you to be a student from any of the above. It therefore makes sense to look through the course material and decide which best suits your needs and interests.

Typical Master's degree

While there are a large number of courses available from a range of organisations, local universities or undergraduate departments a key question is: what is the core knowledge that every educator should have to undertake the role? It is perhaps worth looking at the content of a Master's course in Medical Education which usually comprises a Certificate, a Diploma and then a thesis for the final award of the degree. The good point about this approach is that it gives you stop-off points and allows you to complete it at your own pace. The courses are designed to be relevant to the delivery of education in the workplace and specific to medical education.

Typically you will undertake core modules eg:

- Learning and teaching in medical education
- Principles of assessment in medical education
- Leadership in healthcare and healthcare education
- Curriculum planning and evaluation
- Medical education research

These modules typically form the backbone of the Certificate work but are supplemented with optional modules which can be chosen depending on personal interest eg:

- Clinical skills and simulation for education and practice
- Technology-enhanced learning
- Assessment, knowledge, skills and attitudes
- Clinical teaching
- Education support and resilience
- Faculty development and health professions

The above areas are commonly assessed via a written assignment. The Certificate (60 credits) will equip practitioners to be teachers with a solid grounding in a pedagogical and evidence-based approach. You need to undertake three 20-credit modules of which usually two need to be core, plus one optional module.

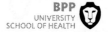

The Diploma requires a further 60 credits. This is one core module and two optional modules; however, if you want to progress to the Master's phase then you would need to have research in medical education as one of the modules.

Finally the dissertation (a further 60 credits) will equip you to use diverse methodologies to explore an innovative and original question. Typically this is 12,000–15,000 words to obtain your Master's degree.

A Master's degree may not be what you want to focus on but the stepwise progression from Certificate through to Diploma will unquestionably give you a very solid platform for your day to day teaching. It also enables you to fund each section separately thus spreading the costs.

If your interest is sufficiently piqued you may decide that you wish to undertake further research in medical education and study for a PhD. In many ways this is for the individual who wants to peruse an academic career within the university setting. This will take a minimum of three years researching into a given field in medical education that particularly interests you. Funding may be available not only from the university department but also from outside agencies and the medical education organisations that look to invest their charitable funds for the advance of the study of medical education. You are making a definite career decision by undertaking a PhD and aligning yourself to a university department but it is still possible to continue to undertake clinical work at the same time.

Case study

I decided to undertake a Master's degree to improve my understanding of both medical education and teaching but also I felt that without showing a commitment to medical education future jobs may well be out of reach. I was in General Practice at the time and the only practical way of undertaking the study was to do a distance learning package. I applied to the Deanery for funding and they were happy to support my application. I started the Dundee course and they sent all the paperwork required to complete the assignments. Indeed the written material they supplied was very comprehensive. I started it in the summer and at the time my daughter sailed every Saturday morning. I used to drop her at the club and would bring all my reading materials for each assignment. At the end of the morning I would have completed the required reading and I would then get up on Sunday morning to begin writing. I followed this same pattern for all my assignments through to the diploma.

When it came to undertaking the dissertation I needed to do an extensive literature search. I personally felt I needed protected time to do this and to start writing. I therefore took two weeks' annual leave to kick-start the process. This worked well and I took a further two weeks later in the year to complete the task. I was awarded my Master's and went on to have a career in medical education away from primary care.

2. **University internal programmes**

If you work in the university setting perhaps having taken a lectureship role to combine with your clinical work you will find that the university offers an induction programme that includes knowledge and skills for teaching. While the programmes can vary from university to university and some are not compulsory you can gain a great deal from being involved in this free(!) programme.

The Higher Education Academy (HEA) is the organisation that promotes and indeed sets the standards for educational excellence in the university setting. These standards are not specific for medical education but are generic and pertinent to all disciplines. The HEA aims to raise the profile of teaching so staff are recognised for their work and are motivated to keep developing their knowledge and careers. They use the UK professional standards framework which is a comprehensive set of professional standards and guidelines for everyone involved in teaching and supporting learners. This framework has similarities to that used by the GMC for its standards for medical educators.

There is also the opportunity to become a Fellow of the HEA which brings a range of benefits (not just the post-nominal

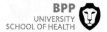

FHEA!). It helps consolidate personal development as a teacher, demonstrating a commitment to teaching through engagement in a practical process that encourages research, reflection and development. So again this avenue is open to those who are developing their education careers in the higher education setting and is recognised extensively in the sector.

Applications are from individuals who must complete an extensive application process comprising:

- Section one. A list of learning and teaching/CPD activities mapped against the appropriate areas of activity, core knowledge and professional values.

- Section two. A reflective account of practice on the areas of:

  - Design and plan learning activities and/or programmes of study, teaching and/or support learning

  - Assess and give feedback to learners

  - Develop effective learning environments and approaches to student support and guidance

  - Engage in CPD in subjects/disciplines and their pedagogy, incorporating research, scholarship and the evaluation of professional practice

Completing the above and adding your referees will enable you to apply to become a Fellow of the HEA and again boost your standing in education.

3. **Royal Colleges**

The Royal College of Physicians (RCP) has designed a Master's in Medical Education (in collaboration with University College London) specifically advertised to meet the requirements of doctors who are intending to have a significant role in medical education.

The programme is designed with Certificate and Diploma levels, each with four modules. Each module has a focus on teaching and learning in a clinical setting. There are face to face days with each module, so there is that to account for. In the last year the dissertation focuses on a piece of research on any aspect of medical education. Examples of previous dissertations can be seen on the RCP Medical Education Resource Centre pages.

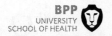

So, it is important to choose the right course for your future needs and career aspirations. Remember someone will have to pay the fees (and that might be you!) which are at least £9,000 for the entire course.

Case study

As a new principal in General Practice I was clear from the start (indeed I mentioned it at my interview!) that I wanted to be a GP trainer. This required the permission of all my partners in the first instance. Fortunately the practice was already a training practice and the current training was moving on to be the local vocational training scheme course organiser. It therefore fitted nicely to have a second qualified trainer in the practice. Within the region there was a three-day residential course which comprised of attendance at three courses over the space of a year. The course was also registered with the local university to award a certificate in medical education at the end of the process. Written work and a portfolio had to be undertaken to underpin the course and these were then marked independently by the university to award the certificate in medical education. This, however, did not yet make you qualified to train within the region. A further inspection visit to the practice was required. This ensured that the practice demonstrated the appropriate standards to be a training practice and my own consultations and teaching were also reviewed on video on the day. Following that inspection process (and having been awarded the Certificate) I was recommended to have my first trainee. While the practice picked up the residential fees and certificate fees I still had to do the work! Fitting the work into my spare time was less onerous than I first thought (but then you would have to ask my partner!) as the work was relevant and practical. It is worth noting that not every region in the UK requires a certificate to become a GP trainer so it is certainly worth enquiring with your GP Director about the local rules and regulations.

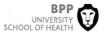

Barriers

When considering embarking on further CPD or formal qualifications in medical education or related areas you will need to reflect on some barriers that you will have to manage to be successful in your study. These include:

- Time
- Money
- Commitment
- Support

The process is very similar to studying for your college exams. You have to give the time, pay the fees, knuckle down and hopefully have sufficient support at work and at home to be successful. The major difference between this and your professional exams is that it is essentially voluntary. While the new GMC standards for Educational Supervisors are essentially mandatory, further development of an educational portfolio is not. So ultimately the major barrier to advancing your career and knowledge is yourself!

Drivers

The status of medical education has been boosted over the last few years. This is due to several factors, all of which have had a positive effect in the workplace.

Appraisal and revalidation, whatever else they are designed to achieve, have ensured that the job plan must have protected time for those in an educational role. The appraisal process allows the individual to focus on their developmental needs for all aspects of their working week, including educational delivery. You are being paid to deliver education and therefore it has a new value to the organisation and they have a right to hold educators to account for that investment.

The GMC educator standards as already mentioned are mandatory and each NHS organisation needs to ensure that it complies with these standards. The fact that the hospitals with the best training standards also produce the best patient outcomes has been known for a long time and again should be a major driver for any Chief Executive in their investment in education strategy.

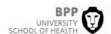

The number of educational roles that are now advertised has seen an increase in recent years to help train the doctors to pass their exams, to undertake quality improvement projects and to undertake research and publish. This allows individuals to see a potential career pathway in medical education which is separate from their clinical commitment. More and more doctors are looking to establish portfolio careers and medical education lends itself very well in fulfilling this agenda.

Who can help?

There are any number of people and organisations that can offer advice on furthering your career in medical education. First stop is to just ask the person doing the job you would like to train towards. So any of the following within your working environment:

- Lecturer
- Senior Lecturer
- College Tutor
- Course Organiser
- GP Trainer
- Associate Dean
- Researcher in Medical Education
- GP Director
- Director of Medical Education
- Postgraduate Dean
- Undergraduate Dean

All the above would be happy to discuss your career aspirations and some would be able to let to you know of potential vacancies going forward.

There are a number of medical education organisations that you may also wish to sound out or indeed join and these can again lead you to look at different aspects of the field of medical education:

- Association for the Study of Medical Education was established in 1957 and aims to help meet the needs of teachers, trainers and learners across medical education by supporting research-informed best practice. Its membership focuses on all who are involved in medical education and training in the UK and it provides CPD, leadership development and research in medical education networks.

- Association for Medical Education in Europe, founded in 1972, aims to promote excellence in education in healthcare professions across a broad spectrum. It is a worldwide organisation with members across 90 countries.

- Academy of Medical Educators was established in 2006 as a multiprofessional organisation with the aim of providing leadership and promoting standards in medical education. It has developed the professional standards that formed the backbone of those adopted by the GMC.

- National Association of Clinical Tutors UK (NACT UK). NACT UK was formed in 1969 with the aim to support and represent local leaders who deliver medical and dental education across the UK.

- Association for Simulated Practice in Healthcare is dedicated to improving patient care and professional performance by the use of simulated practice and technology-enhanced learning.

All the above organisations are there to support those undertaking roles in medical education and you may benefit greatly from joining one that is most closely related to the job you are undertaking or going to undertake. All these organisations run conferences during the year and can fulfil your CPD needs. They have active websites with a great deal of useful information, not just about the courses but also educational materials that you would find useful. They are also a great opportunity to network with other medical educators and share ideas and best practice.

In addition, the Faculty of Medical Leadership and Management (FMLM) is a useful organisation to get involved in. In any medical education role you will have leadership responsibilities and the FMLM was established in 2011 to support doctors in such leadership roles.

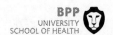

Other relevant qualifications

The other degree that you might want to consider undertaking is a Master's in Business Administration (MBA). This may seem rather strange for those involved in medical education but it could prove very valuable for those that go on to undertake substantive roles in the education management arena eg GP Director, Postgraduate Dean or Medical Director. While you will learn a great deal in undertaking the Certificate and Diploma in Medical Education, this will be of great help to all those that are involved in day to day delivery of education in the workplace. When you climb the ladder to more substantive roles a larger part of your time will be dealing with the administrative delivery of education, budgets and with meetings and people. Skills learnt by undertaking an MBA could give you a valuable insight into how to deliver organisational goals and think through the wider strategic aims of the organisation.

Case study

As a Postgraduate Dean I encouraged all my senior team members to undertake the steps towards a Master's in medical education. I was able to fund their fees on a stepwise progression from certificate through to diploma and Master's thesis. This spread the costs over several years. For the first four to five years most were delighted to be given the opportunity and signed up and progressed. However, after this time and as new members joined the team there was a shift in thinking. While I continued to offer the fees for the Master's in medical education new recruits asked if they could do an MBA instead. I was happy to agree and the knowledge they acquired brought a new dimension to the running of the Deanery, placing it much more on a fit for purpose organisational structure delivering medical education.

Chapter summary

It is important that whatever institute you belong to you fulfil the basic criteria for all medical educators as defined by the GMC's new standards. From there you can undertake local courses that may be mandatory within the undergraduate sector as an induction programme or go to more formal accredited courses. It remains unlikely that the more senior jobs in education will be available to anyone who has not shown some commitment to undertaking these formal routes as interviewers do look for an objective measure of interest from the candidate. It is therefore up to you to decide exactly how much and how far you wish to develop and invest in a medical education portfolio or career.

Key points

- Think what career you want to have: portfolio or full time.
- Look and see who is doing the job you would like to do.
- Speak to senior educators to let them know your interest.
- Look to undertake further qualifications in medical education.
- Ask if funding is available.
- Ensure you have protected time in the job plan for education.
- Use the appraisal process to engage the trust in your CPD requirements for medical education.
- Join one of the medical associations for further support and CPD guidance.
- Keep applying for posts. You will get noticed.
- Enjoy the journey.

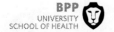
BPP
UNIVERSITY
SCHOOL OF HEALTH

Useful resources

Association for the Study of Medical Education – www.asme.org.uk/

Academy of Medical Educators – www.medicaleducators.org

Association for Simulated Practice in Healthcare – www.aspih. org.uk/

Faculty of Medical Leadership and Management – www.fmlm.ac.uk

Higher Education Academy – www.heacademy.ac.uk

National Association of Clinical Tutors – www.nact.org.uk/

PRINCE2 Foundation and Practitioner online learning – www. prince2.com/uk/training/prince2/foundation-practitioner/online

Royal College of Physicians website for educators – www.rcplondon. ac.uk/education-practice/courses/msc-medical-education

References

Academy of Medical Educators (2014) *Professional Standards for Medical, Dental and Veterinary Educators*. Cardiff: Academy of Medical Educators.

Deming, WE (1983) *Out of the Crisis*. Cambridge, MA: Massachusetts Institute of Technology Centre for Advanced Engineering Study.

General Medical Council (2013) *Good Medical Practice*. [Online]. Available at: www.gmc-uk.org/guidance/good_medical_practice. asp [Accessed 21 June 2017].

General Medical Council (2015) *Promoting Excellence: Standards for Medical Education and Training*. [Online]. Available at: www.gmc-uk.org/education/standards.asp [Accessed 21 June 2017].

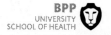

Chapter 7

Current frameworks in medical education

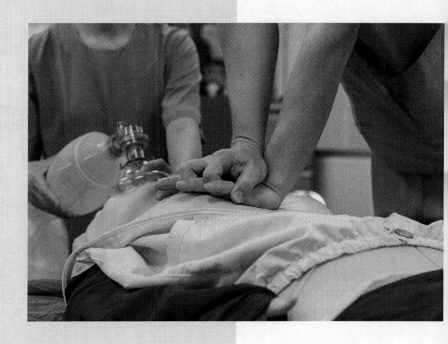

Introduction

Medical educators work within a given framework to deliver the best possible training for the best patient outcomes. As a medical educator the framework in which you will operate comes from many sources, some of which are in statute and others are guidance for best practice. It is essential that as a medical educator you have an understanding of the non-negotiable elements that every medical student and trainee has to adhere to and fulfil in order to progress in their training and gain the ultimate award of a Certificate of Completion of Training.

It is also important to be up to date with the latest changes to both the General Medical Council (GMC) requirements and curriculum requirements. Both are reviewed on a regular, even, ongoing basis.

It is worth first considering the changes that the GMC has introduced to unify the standards across undergraduate and postgraduate education. These have already been mentioned in Chapter 6 however they need to be seen in the whole as a driver for improving education and patient care. In addition, if you are in an NHS medical education role it is important to understand the strategic needs of the organisation and the process of revalidation and related continuing professional development (CPD).

General Medical Council (GMC) role in education and training

The GMC has two major roles. The first is the regulation of doctors and the second is setting standards for education and training of medical students and trainee doctors.

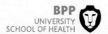

Stage	Selection into medical school	Medical school years	Foundation training	Specialty training
Image	Selection into medical school	Medical school years	Foundation training	Specialty training
Context	Around 100,000 applicants apply for a place at medical school each year. Only around 6,000 are chosen.	There are 41,000 medical students at the UK's 31 medical schools. Degree courses last between four and six years.	The Foundation Programme is a two year training programme for doctors after leaving medical school. There are around 15,000 doctors on the programme currently.	After Foundation training most doctors enter specialty training. There are over 100 specialties and sub-specialty courses. There are around 40,000 doctors doing speciality or GP training in the UK.
Our role	We set the standards that medical schools have to meet. We say selection methods must be 'open, objective and fair'.	We set the standards around the education medical students receive. • These include: the standards medical schools must meet in teaching and assessing students • the skills and behaviours students must have learned to complete the course. We monitor and check to make sure these standards are maintained. Ultimately it's our job to decide if a university should be allowed to issue medical degrees.	We set the standards for the programme, including the level the doctor must reach by the end of the two years, and we approve the curriculum. We monitor and check to make sure the standards we set are maintained.	We set the standards which training organisations must meet, and the standards that doctors in training must reach by the end of training. Our role includes approving the curricula for each training programme. We monitor and check to make sure the standards we set are maintained. One way we do this is by conducting a comprehensive survey of all doctors in training each year.
The role of others	Empty cell	Medical schools set the curricula and provide the education to medical students. Degree courses last between four and six years.	Medical graduates have to apply to regional postgraduate training bodies called deaneries – or in England, local education training boards (LETBs). They co-ordinate, supervise and monitor individual doctors' progress. The curriculum for the Foundation Programme is developed by the Academy of Medical Royal Colleges.	The UK's Medical Royal Colleges and Faculties set the curriculum for specialty and GP training courses. Deaneries and LETBs manage the delivery of specialty training. Trainees receive training at approved hospitals, clinics and GP surgeries.

Figure 7.1 The key roles of the General Medical Council (GMC, 2017)

Figure 7.1 reflects the roles that the GMC undertakes in both undergraduate and postgraduate education. You will need to understand these if involved with delivering education as ultimately you may be responsible to the regulator for the quality management of the process. The GMC has also now combined its

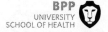

visiting process and looks at both medical schools and Postgraduate Deaneries within a geographical area and how they work together across the institutions. All those involved in educational delivery, from the Educational Supervisors (ESs) and lecturers up to the Undergraduate and Postgraduate Deans will potentially be interviewed and need to show an understanding of the cross-collaboration and the strategic direction of education within the locality. The GMC will also explore the level of engagement of learners, medical students and trainees with the medical school and Postgraduate Deanery. This clearly brings to the fore the lines of communication from ESs and undergraduate tutors/lecturers through to the central education teams. How much a part of the educational infrastructure individuals feel part of, how they can raise concerns, what feedback and support they get and how the trainees feel part of the collective are central to the functioning of the educational environment in which education and training operates. The GMC will comment on all these aspects at their visits and will look for evidence of best practice which they will disseminate across the UK.

Locality visits tend to be on a five-year cycle but if issues are found or raised at a visit then follow-up visits will continue until a suitable resolution is found to move forward. As yet no medical school has been deemed to be below the level at which it would be refused approval to teach. However, the newer medical schools have had reviews of their curricula that have meant they need more time for full approval to be issued. The newer private medical schools are also asked to 'buddy up' with an established local medical school to help them through the approvals process.

No Postgraduate Deanery has ever been closed but if serious patient safety issues are identified trainees have been relocated from repeatedly underperforming departments. This should have already been on the Deanery radar and it is likely that they will have asked the GMC to visit to approve their recommendation of moving trainees. Objective evidence is required to ensure an open and transparent process with these sensitive issues. It should also not have come as a shock to the department or Trust/Health Board which means prior warnings and visits will have been undertaken. These visits come under the quality management process of each Deanery. Typically, these are risk-based escalation processes.

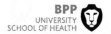

GMC education and training standards

The GMC document *Promoting Excellence: Standards for Medical Education and Training* (GMC, 2015) sets out the ten standards that are expected from organisations responsible for education and training medical students and doctors in the UK. These standards are an update and replace *Tomorrow's Doctors* (2009), the previous standards for undergraduate education, and *The Trainee Doctor* (2011) which stated the standards for postgraduate training. The new standards go across both the undergraduate and postgraduate fields which is a major step forward in the unification of what is expected. It is also a great help in the workplace; as is frequently the case, you will be responsible for education across undergraduate and postgraduate.

The GMC's ten standards are arranged in five themes as follows.

Theme 1. Learning environment and culture

This theme is concerned with the learning environment and the focus is on both the learner's and teacher's needs. There are specific requirements on each of the Local Education Providers (LEPs) to ensure there are processes in place that provide a culture that genuinely supports education and learning. So for example requirement R1.4 states:

> *Organisations must demonstrate a learning environment and culture that supports learners to be open and honest with patients when things go wrong – known as their professional duty of candour – and help them to develop the skills to communicate with tact, sensitivity and empathy.*

This means that LEPs have to have governance processes in place to ensure that any concerns raised are escalated to the board so that action can be taken. In order for this to happen LEPs need to work closely with the local Postgraduate Deanery and medical schools to develop and maintain an educationally rich environment. It is clear that if there is a positive learning environment for medical students and trainees there is likely to be a similar positive experience for all other healthcare learners.

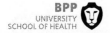
BPP
UNIVERSITY
SCHOOL OF HEALTH

Theme 2. Educational governance and leadership

This theme is about having the infrastructure and support to treat learners according to the principles of safety, equality and fairness. The organisation should therefore integrate educational and clinical governance to keep patients and learners safe and create an appropriate learning environment and organisational culture.

Theme 3. Supporting learners

This theme was covered in more depth in Chapter 6 and the focus is on ensuring that learners get effective educational and pastoral support, so they can demonstrate what is expected in 'good medical practice' and achieve the learning outcomes required by their curriculum.

Theme 4. Supporting educators

The importance of this theme is the cornerstone of educational delivery. The educators have to have the necessary knowledge and skills for the role and get the support and resources they need to deliver effective education and training. This is the final step in truly professionalising the role of the educator. The specific roles covered by this are:

- Those that oversee medical students' progress at each medical school

- Lead co-ordinators for undergraduate education at each LEP

- Named ESs

- Named clinical supervisors

Medical trainers in the four specific roles above are responsible for complying with the arrangements set out by medical schools and Postgraduate Deans to meet GMC requirements for recognising and approving trainers. Furthermore, the LEP will be held to account for the production of a list of these trainers and the educational support and time provided for them to undertake the role.

Theme 5. Developing and implementing curricula and assessments

The GMC has a statutory responsibility to regulate curricula and assessments according to the stages of training. The GMC sets the learning outcomes required of medical students when they graduate

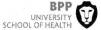

and the standards that medical schools must meet when teaching, assessing and providing learning opportunities for the students.

Royal Colleges, faculties and specialty associations develop postgraduate curricula including assessment strategies and again the GMC approves them against the standards for curricula and assessment systems.

It will always be important that the ES is aware of any changes or indeed potential changes to the curriculum that may occur and communicate these to the trainee. Gone are the days that a trainee could remain on the curriculum that was in place when they started and they will need to know the modifications that are required to proceed on to their Certificate of Completion of Training (CCT). These modifications will be a response to updates in the knowledge base, introduction of new medication or therapies, changing patient pathways or workforce planning.

It is essential that those involved in medical education understand the above criteria and how they need to be implemented in the workplace. At one level these new standards are a great step forward helping to produce the learning environments that medical students and trainees will thrive in. At an organisational level failure to adhere to these standards potentially risks the status of the LEP as a place to learn and train.

Revalidation

As a General Practitioner, Consultant or Staff/Associate Specialist grade in the UK, if you have any education roles these should be a part of the discussion at your annual appraisal and hence support your revalidation. The GMC expects that you will reflect on all aspects of your roles – clinical, education, research etc – and ensure that you have evidence that you are up to date (see Chapter 6).

The GMC introduced revalidation and relicensing for all doctors in the UK in 2012. This process is in a five-year cycle and is there to reassure the public that the doctor they are seeing is up to date and has a licence to practise in good standing with the regulator. The guidance provided sets out the supporting information that is required at the annual appraisal and falls into four broad categories:

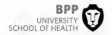

1. General information – providing context about what you do in all aspects of your work

2. Keeping up to date – maintaining and enhancing the quality of your professional work

3. Review of your practice – evaluating the quality of your professional work

4. Feedback on your practice – how others perceive the quality of your professional work

From this there are six types of supporting information that you will be expected to show and discuss at the appraisal at least once per five-year cycle.

1. CPD for all roles

2. Quality improvement activity

3. Significant events

4. Feedback from colleagues

5. Feedback from patients

6. Review of complaints and compliments within the portfolio but to reflect and comment on all aspects of the work you undertake and what you might want to do differently in the future

This process includes the doctors in training and currently the cycle starts at registration. The trainee has an Annual Review of Competency Progression (ARCP), an appraisal process underpinned by their portfolio which has to be up to date. Little more is required for them to get their yearly sign-off for the revalidation process and five years' worth of the reviews will be sufficient evidence that they fulfil the GMC requirements. The GMC is reviewing the whole process but since not everyone will have been through the cycle until 2018 we can expect little changes currently.

The positive aspects of revalidation are the reflective nature of the process which ensure the individual must review and reflect on all aspects of their work and CPD. A positive development is the 360 degree feedback from colleagues that you work with and your reflections on what you will change based on that feedback. The mandatory nature of the appraisal process (which had been

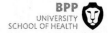

patchy previously) is again a positive move forward. It is easiest done if the individual fills in the forms as they go along rather than waiting to gather all the evidence just prior to their yearly appraisal. It does remain an administrative burden for the individual and it will be interesting to see what changes the GMC will make to the process when the first cycle has been reviewed. If the aim is to give the public reassurance of the good standing of the doctor then the validity of some aspects of the process may well become redundant.

The role of the ES is to undertake the yearly appraisal and ensure that the trainee fully understands the revalidation concept and gets them fully engaged as it will be there for their professional life. The whole system is simpler for the trainee as the processes are already in place for them to collect the information and undergo the yearly appraisal process. The Responsible Officer for the trainee is the Postgraduate Dean and when the paperwork has been agreed with the trainee and ES the Dean is in a position to make a recommendation to the GMC for the relicensing/revalidation process. It is the GMC that has the authority to authorise the process and set the next date in the cycle.

Continuing professional development (CPD)

The GMC standards are now explicit in that everyone with educational/training roles has to demonstrate that they are keeping up to date with their role as an educator. This must be clearly articulated at the yearly appraisal and job planning process and supported by the LEP. It is an essential element of the revalidation and relicensing process. Good medical practice requires all doctors to keep their knowledge and skills up to date, encouraging them to take part in educational activity that maintain and further develop their clinical skills and knowledge. In discussing this at the appraisal consideration should be given to the following:

- Personal learning. Your own professional learning needs within the context of patients' needs and those of the service.

- Scope of practice. It should cover the breadth of the professional activities you undertake in the role.

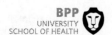

- Outcomes. What output the activity has on impact and improvement of performance.

- Needs based. This is about your current scope of practice and also how it will develop going forward.

- Appraisal and clinical governance. You need to comment on how you participate in clinical governance processes and how they shed light on your professional and work practices.

Logging the activity in your appraisal portfolio is the simplest way of keeping track and being able to reflect on the merits or otherwise of the educational CPD. Reviewing your 360 degree feedback can also help in identifying the areas of practice that you may need to work on or improve. While most of the Royal Colleges have a fixed number of hours of CPD that clinicians should undertake each year, there is no fixed rate for educators. Your learning therefore needs planning and consideration of the available opportunities that are provided. It is common for your local Postgraduate Deanery and medical school to host several educator updates each year and this can certainly help you to keep you abreast of any new changes to the regulatory framework. Developing as an educator can involve undertaking a higher degree and this would certainly fulfil all your CPD requirements, possibly for several years.

Registration

On passing finals a medical student applies to the GMC for provisional registration. This is required to start a job as a Foundation Year 1 doctor in the UK. At the end of that first year the individual is eligible to apply for full registration. They will have had to demonstrate the competencies required in the foundation curriculum, have an up to date portfolio and had an appraisal. Foundation Year 1 doctors can only work in an educationally approved (by the GMC) post and cannot undertake any locum work or work in any position that is for a fully registered doctor. This restricts them to an approved Foundation Year 1 rotation which in times of undersubscription to the Foundation Programme is not a problem but, with increases to the number of medical students in England, the potential removal of the cap on overseas students and the rise of private UK-based medical schools, this may not always be the case. Without full registration the individual cannot

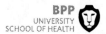

work and the only current method of getting that is satisfactory completion of the Foundation Year 1. Issues around moving the point of registration and a national Medical Licensing Assessment will be covered in Chapter 9 but could have a profound effect on the postgraduate educational landscape.

Less than full time training

There is an increasing number of trainees that wish to work less than full time (LTFT) and this trend shows no sign of doing anything other than increasing. While the focus in all the curricula has been on a competency-based framework, very few trainees have actually managed (or indeed wanted!) to reduce the length of time taken to train. The GMC issued new guidance in October 2011 to clarify both the rules and the European Union (EU) legislation. It had been the rule that LTFT were expected to work a minimum of 50% of full time; however, the EU discontinued this and there is actually no legislation on the minimum time proportion. Article 22 of the EU directive permits member states to authorise part-time training under conditions laid down by the competent authority, that authority in the UK being the GMC. After consultation with key interested parties the GMC issued guidance which agrees an enforceable minimum of 50% with flexibility to reduce to 20% in exceptional circumstances. Any time less than the 50% minimum must be agreed with the responsible Postgraduate Dean and should only be for a maximum of 12 months and subject to regular reviews. In terms of training and the role of the ES, they need to ensure that the LTFT complies with the working hours but has access to all aspects of the curriculum and the breadth and depth of the clinical experience commensurate with the available hours. This does mean full access to the teaching sessions on the days worked. The ES needs to ensure that a realistic educational plan is in place at the start of any year with goals that are achievable and regularly reviewed. The trainee needs to be aware of any changes to the curriculum that occur and the rules regarding the need to change to the new curriculum. This is particularly important as the trainee needs to be up to date with changes that affect patient care and reflect best-known practice. Because of the potential length of time an LTFT takes it can be easy to be out of date.

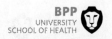

The recent changes to the contract for junior doctors in England have revealed much dissatisfaction on the lack of flexibility with training and the Secretary of State asked the GMC to review the lack of flexibility in the system and not just the LTFT issue. The GMC proposed a seven point plan specifically geared to delivering more flexibility.

- Training will be organised by outcomes rather than time spent in training.

- Related specialties curricula will share common outcomes and elements.

- The GMC will reduce the burden of its approval system so that medical colleges and faculties can make changes to the postgraduate curricula more quickly.

- The GMC will work with others to promote mechanisms which already exist to help trainees change training programmes.

- The GMC will ask the Government to make the law less restrictive so that it can be more agile in approving training.

- The GMC will support doctors with specific capabilities or needs.

- The GMC will encourage national educational bodies to continue to focus on work–life balance of trainees.

The above will place an added responsibility on all ESs, Training Programme Directors (TPDs), Heads of Specialty School and the ARCP process. A better understanding of the competencies that are common between specialties, moving to a truly outcomes-based training pathway and the whole concept of generic professional capabilities will require the entire medical education team to understand them and put them into practice with the trainee.

Generic professional capabilities (GPCs)

The GMC has altered the way it responds to the curricula and the whole skill set it expects doctors to have developed and demonstrate by the time they achieve their CCT. Previous specialty curricula could be considered to be in silos, with individual skills passed (or failed) without reference to a more holistic approach to the patient. This reductionist approach has perhaps engendered the

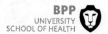

lack of common skills across the specialties and the wider patient focus rather than disease focus approach to healthcare. The GPCs are an articulation of the 'put the patient first' ethos and what is required to work in a modern multiprofessional NHS.

These, therefore, are broader skills needed by doctors to help provide safe and effective patient care and are therefore common to all doctors across all specialties.

This is clearly a further role that the ESs, TPDs and the wider Postgraduate Deanery will have to undertake to ensure that each trainee has the requisite generic skills for the job.

The GMC has been working closely with all the Royal Colleges on developing guidance to embed the GPCs into the curricula. This will then translate down into the workplace for support to:

- Integrate the GPCs framework into curricula and assessment processes
- Identify the required levels of capability for each domain across all medical specialties
- Identify appropriate assessment methods

Generic professional capabilities (GPCs) are broader human skills, such as communication and team working, needed by doctors to help provide safe and effective patient care. They are common to doctors across all medical specialities.

We are working jointly with the Academy of Medical Royal Colleges (Academy) to help medical royal colleges and faculties embed generic professional capabilities into all postgraduate medical curricula in 2017.

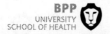

GPC framework

The GPC framework is a matrix of educational outcomes that describe essential and critical capabilities underpinning core professional practice in the United Kingdom.

The framework has nine domains. All domains are interdependent and all are important.

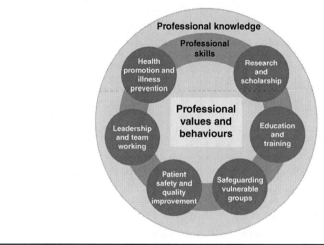

Figure 7.2 Generic Professional Capabilities (GMC, 2017)

Figure 7.2 demonstrates the breadth and depth of what is required to fulfil the GPCs and its contribution to the overall CCT. New assessment tools and embedding skills that can be difficult to define at various points in training will all be required of the educational and clinical supervisor to fully report at the yearly ARCP. It goes without saying that the ESs and TPDs should be able to demonstrate all the requisite skills and indeed be a role model for the trainee. Looking at some of these skills such as team working and leadership, which cover a wide range of experiences within the workplace, the assessment of them can be difficult. The ES should not have a reductionist approach to the sign-off of these skills as information on the trainee's performance must be sourced from different avenues and people. The crux for the ES is therefore not when they have a sense that the trainee actually does perform these skills at the appropriate level but what to do when they fall short of the standard. If the trainee is to have their training extended because they have not demonstrated a skill they will need an educational prescription which should outline:

- The area that needs further work

- The time frame to demonstrate gaining the competence

- The support the trainee can expect to receive

- Any additional help or courses that would be appropriate to undertake

- An explicit understanding of the assessment during the remedial period

This is an outline of what the trainee should expect from the process and does make the process legally defendable. Clear instructions and documentation will be required if the trainee is ultimately to be removed from training and will be necessary for any potential inevitable appeal. However, in helping the trainee to get back on track the better the educational prescription, the easier the task for trainee and trainer alike.

Credentials

The GMC was aware of several areas of practice that were in fact unregulated. This clearly posed a threat to patient safety as doctors could undertake work or procedures that are outside the normal training pathway and curricula approved by the GMC. Examples of these are Musculoskeletal Medicine, Breast Disease Management and Forensic Medicine. The GMC has therefore sought to introduce the concept of a credential. This would involve the Faculty currently delivering the subject matter to submit a curricula for approval to the GMC. It should contain an appropriate assessment methodology, be sponsored by a credible organisation and cover a clinical area of practice that the public are in need of. Following the approval of the curricula those doctors that fulfil the criteria and have been properly assessed would be granted a credential in the subject. This qualification would appear on the medical register beside their name. This would give the public reassurance that the doctor was qualified in the given field. These new curricula may have to be overseen by the local Postgraduate Deanery using the same clinical governance procedures in place for any other specialty. The nature of the credential may mean that not every LEP will necessarily have the clinical material or be able to provide the breadth and depth

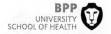

of what would be required to fulfil the curricula. The delivery of a specific credential may therefore be patchy around the country and will be related to those also currently undertaking the specialty and therefore able to supervise new trainees.

The 'Shape of Training' report by Professor David Greenaway also looked at introducing credentials and caused some confusion with the original GMC undertaking of just the unregulated areas of practice. The original 'Shape' report was designed to look at all aspects of postgraduate training and specifically what steps need to be taken to introduce more generalist training. Within its 19 recommendations it mentioned credentials as a means of undertaking sub-specialty training after obtaining a generalist certificate in the specialty. In this model the sub-specialty curricula and assessments would be taken out of the generalist curriculum and operate as a standalone qualification. The timing of this as to whether it still could occur in the generalist training period or has to be after the completion of the certificate of generalist training may well vary. The positives about this model is that it produces more doctors with a generalist skill set able to provide triage at the front door of a hospital and provide a more holistic approach for the patient. It could also be much more responsive to workforce planning and demands for tertiary service skills. New credentials could be put in place that responded to local health needs of the population. As yet there is no agreement on the way forward on the generalist agenda or the thorny issue of who might pay for the training of the doctors looking to undertake the credential or sub-specialty. However, there remains a great deal of interest in the concept, particularly in the light of the many and varied fellowships that are currently being offered to provide additional skills to senior trainees and new consultants. Interest is also high in the health administrations as they seek to produce new models of healthcare and be responsive to local issues (eg rural health). When credentials move forward the process will certainly change the training landscape. More hospitals will be training those for the generalist curricula in the specialty and potentially fewer hospitals will train for sub-specialty credentials.

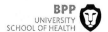

Chapter summary

The role of those involved in the delivery of medical education is underpinned by regulations and standards. These can be fast changing and require additional training for all in medical education roles and the trainees so they can be fully understood and complied with. The effect of new contracts on working and the training environment should not be underestimated. Keeping up to date is required by all involved in medical education and forms part of the normal CPD expected for revalidation and relicensing.

Key points

- Use CPD to keep up to date with new standards and curricula updates.

- Check GMC website for potential changes to regulations.

- Be aware of political impacts on contracts and knock-on effects to training.

- Keep medical students and trainees informed of any changes.

- Check what courses your local Deanery or medical school are delivering as it will be related to changes in educational delivery.

- Join a medical education group that relates best to your day to day work.

Useful resources

General Medical Council Generic Professional Capabilities framework – www.gmc-uk.org/education/postgraduate/GPC.asp

References

General Medical Council (2013) *Good Medical Practice*. [Online]. Available at: www.gmc-uk.org/guidance/good_medical_practice.asp [Accessed 21 June 2017].

General Medical Council (2015) *Outcomes for Graduates*. [Online]. Available at: www.gmc-uk.org/education/undergraduate/undergrad_outcomes.asp [Accessed 21 June 2017].

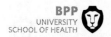

General Medical Council (2015) *Promoting Excellence: Standards for Medical Education and Training*. [Online]. Available at: www.gmc-uk.org/education/standards.asp [Accessed 21 June 2017].

General Medical Council (2012) *Recognising and Approving Trainers: the Implementation Plan*. [Online]. Available at: www.gmc-uk.org/Approving_trainers_implementation_plan_Aug_12.pdf_56452109.pdf [Accessed 21 June 2017].

General Medical Council (2010) *Standards for Curricula and Assessment Systems*. [Online]. Available at: www.gmc-uk.org/6___PMETB_Merger___Governance_Standards_and_Policies___Annex_C.pdf_36034678.pdf [Accessed 21 June 2017].

Greenaway, D (2013) *Shape of Training: Securing the future of excellent patient care – the final report of the independent review*. [Online]. Available at: www.shapeoftraining.co.uk/static/documents/content/Shape_of_training_FINAL_Report.pdf_53977887.pdf [Accessed 21 June 2017].

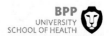

Chapter 8

Surviving as a medical educator

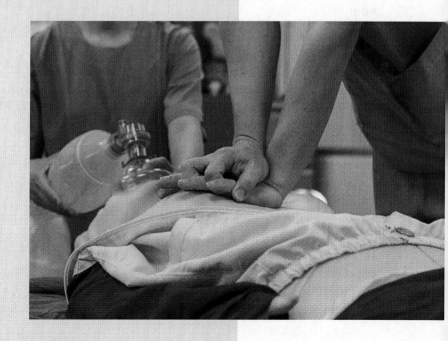

Introduction

In this chapter we will cover a number of specific approaches and models that can at certain points help you to survive and indeed thrive. Clearly it is not just about surviving but rather what steps you can take to ensure your wellbeing.

A number of pillars of wellbeing have been described which include mental health and physical health. It is important for you to recognise very basic health principles and attempt to adhere to them, as it is clear that physical health improves mental health and hence will improve your ability to perform in your role. Simple measures (that clearly aren't that simple) are to maintain a normal weight, low cholesterol and reasonable alcohol intake and to build regular exercise into your weekly routine. It is important for all of us to recognise that when younger we may use physically strenuous de-stressor tactics, such as jogging, cycling, netball, rugby or football. It is a fact of life that as we get older some of these more high impact/high energy sports and physical activities may not be appropriate. It is therefore extremely useful to look ahead at other activities which you may wish to get involved with, recognising that at a certain point you may not be able to pursue previous recreational activities to the same degree as when younger and fitter.

As you move into more senior medical education roles, you hopefully will have acquired the skills to lead an education team irrespective of where that team sits within the hierarchy. Surviving as a doctor and a doctor in medical education will require you to develop skills to manage the pressures and stresses that will arise. Surviving is in large part about knowing yourself. In a medical education role you will interface with a range of stakeholders and staff. There are different pressures from each of these and indeed they too will have their own stresses and pressures to deliver.

There is a useful model to consider within your medical education leadership role, or in fact in any leadership role. This concept recognises that within these roles you will be faced with challenges and you will need to develop skills and resources to cope with these challenges. This balance between skills and challenges has been described as 'the state in which people are so involved in an activity that nothing else seems to matter', which in turn leads to a sense of wellbeing. This model assumes that whenever your skills are at a high level and challenges are high that you will be in a flow channel (this refers to the state of wellbeing) and that if this is out of balance, for example, a low level of skills but high levels of challenges, then the individual will be stressed.

Another useful model is to visualise wellbeing as a seesaw representing the drive of the individual to return to a balanced position. On one side of the seesaw are the challenges, be they social, psychological or physical, and you will face these within your medical education role. On the other side of the seesaw are resources, again social, psychological and physical. So each time you face a challenge this system of resources and challenges is balanced and may come into a state of imbalance and then as an individual you are forced to adapt your resources in order to meet the challenge and become balanced again. This is an interesting model in that it describes wellbeing as a dynamic fluid position as opposed to a particular state.

Individual strategies

We will describe a range of tools and approaches that you can use to help prepare you for the challenges and hence hopefully be able to manage better and feel less stressed and isolated. Not all of these approaches are for everyone and not all are applicable in every situation. Some of these approaches are underpinned by similar concepts and there are overlaps. Some will make more sense to you as an individual and others won't appeal to you. That is fine. The trick is to develop as many tools in your toolbox that work for you.

Resilience

A key concept is resilience, one definition of which is:

> *The ability to rebound from adversity and overcome difficult circumstance* (Carver, 1998)

A lot of us, and you may be like this, thrive whilst working in a challenging and ever-changing environment. But balancing the call of work and family and other demands on our time can be difficult. One constant in healthcare systems is change and this applies equally to the medical education environment.

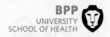

All of the advantages of a portfolio career in medical education discussed in Chapter 2 can lead you to thrive on the challenges but there is a risk of not thriving and therefore it is sensible to develop, use and test out a range of strategies to reduce your risk of burn out.

There are skills you can learn to improve your resilience and deal better under pressure ie to perform better under pressure. One of the first steps is for you to be self-aware, to recognise why you are stressed and to be able to spot the early signs/indicators. So for example, it is useful if you can identify the type of meeting or set of circumstances that can cause you to stress.

Now of course stress is not always bad and you do rely on it as a motivation. The Yerkes-Dodson law (1908) describes the relationship between arousal (stress) and performance. If we see stress as an inner motivating tension the 'good' stress helps you to focus and improves performance. For each individual task there is an optimal level of stress that gives you optimal performance. If stress levels increase past that point then performance drops.

Improving your personal resilience leads to an improvement in performance. There is some discussion about whether training to improve resilience is the best way or is it better to see a range of support systems around you to help prevent stress. Either way, for any one of us having a range of different strategies that we can use at any given circumstance is best.

In a medical education role you will have leadership role/ responsibilities. There is no such thing as the complete leader, ie anyone who has all of the attributes and competencies so part of what you need to do is build a team around you, with your team members having skills, attributes and capabilities that complement yours.

Case study

I had always observed leaders in med education in the medical schools I had worked in and thought that I needed to have all the skills of a leader to do the role. When I became Dean of Medical Education I really worried about what I realised were gaps in my skill set. I was aware that one of the gaps was lack of confidence in direct negotiations and to be frank I had been able to avoid these sorts of situations in

BPP
UNIVERSITY
SCHOOL OF HEALTH

my career up to that point. As Dean I thought that I would have to lead any negotiations and soon after I was appointed there was a proposal to combine the Medical School with the Dental School to create a College. I began to worry about how I would lead these negotiations as the proposal clearly had major implications for the school. Following a couple of team meetings to discuss the plan it was clear to me that some of 'my' team had extensive experience and one non-clinical lecturer had worked for the Advisory, Conciliation and Arbitration Service in a previous role. So I learnt quickly that my role wasn't to be everything to everyone but to lead the team. It wasn't necessarily my role to lead the negotiations but to set out what we needed and empower and support the team who were best placed to negotiate. Once I realised this, the stress reduced significantly as I knew that one of my strengths was seeing the bigger picture and being able to support the staff doing the direct negotiation. What I also learnt was to be aware of the staff's skills and past experiences.

Although as we have said leading effectively is about knowing yourself and being self-aware, you are also required to be very aware of the impact you have on others around you. That can be in your immediate team but also outside of these. This awareness of others has been captured in a number of the concepts including that of emotional intelligence (Goleman, 1996) and is now recognised as a core attribute for any effective leader and this is key in medical education roles. As with any of these models, recent thinking has shifted and describes a mixed model with five main emotional intelligence constructs. These can be a useful reference point for you when reflecting on decisions, upcoming potentially stressful meetings or similar. The five main constructs are:

1. Self-awareness: the ability to recognise and be aware at any moment of your emotions, weaknesses and strengths and recognise your impact on others. This chimes with the concept of mindfulness which in essence is about training yourself to be aware of your thoughts and emotions at any given point. In general we all rush around on the treadmill and don't notice things or pay attention to our own feelings and emotions. The principle of mindfulness is underpinned by the observation

that if we are aware of our feelings and thoughts we can then be aware of how these are driving our behaviour, including decision-making. So getting to a point where you recognise thoughts as mental events can help you from being overwhelmed by those thoughts and associated feelings. So see them as just mental events.

2. Self-regulation: about developing the ability to control your potentially disruptive emotions, such as anger, and redirect that emotion, adapting to the particular circumstances you are in.

3. Social skill: the ability to manage others around you, to help them move in the direction you want or need them to go in.

4. Empathy: the ability to recognise and consider other people's emotions and feelings when you are making decisions.

5. Motivation: having a clear sense of achieving, of delivering.

So emotional intelligence is a form of social intelligence. It is your ability to be aware of your own emotions at any one given moment. High stress meetings are an example, and recognising that how you feel dictates, to a large extent, your actions/behaviour at the meeting.

Case study

One of the most difficult things I had to deliver was reorganising the Training Programme Directors in my specialty school. For years they had worked basically on their own, autonomously, all well-meaning but with no sense of objectives or a consistent approach. So, the Dean told me we needed to reorganise and I did agree but wasn't aware of the enormity of the task. I learnt very quickly that this change was about people, managing people and in particular managing their feelings. The facts are very important but I learnt that by being aware of individuals' feelings and stating that I understood fears helped them to engage with the changes. I made a conscious effort to develop working relationships with the directors. That entailed spending time with them in their working environment and showing that I understood the pressures they were under. It wasn't all plain sailing but managing those relationships at a personal level did help me to be able to reorganise the directors and improve the training to all trainees in my specialty.

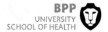

So in any medical education leadership role one trick to surviving and surviving well is to engage with people. Medical education is a people business. So when we engage you must speak to what is important for your audience. One concept that can help you is that there is a certain predictability to people's response to change. These stages were described by Kluber-Ross (1997) and include (in order) the following.

Stage 1. The status quo

At this initial stage people react with shock and denial. This can happen even if you have planned, engaged and communicated the plans. People need time and more information even if they have been given it before. So this is where you being aware of your strengths and weaknesses is important. If communicating the change at the level required is not one of your strengths ensure you have a team of people who have these skills. Directing the team and empowering them to act on your behalf is essential.

Stage 2. Disruption

This stage is referred to as the 'danger zone' for organisations. If this stage isn't handled properly then the whole thing can descend into chaos and you will in all likelihood become more stressed. At this stage people start to react to the change with fear and anger and can actively resist the change. One key thing to bear in mind, to help manage your own stress levels, is that it can appear that some people are reacting negatively 'just to be awkward'. You have to be able to stand back and have a helicopter view. You may not be aware of how the changes you are trying to introduce may actually impact negatively on some staff. Preparing for this stage is crucial and again will help you manage the change and hence achieve your aims.

Stage 3. Exploration

As people begin to accept the change their mindset moves and they start to engage and explore what it means. There is a sense of optimism attached to the change. This is a turning point but acceptance is typically not universal if there is a significant organisational change. Again you have to allow time for staff to explore the 'what's in it for me' question.

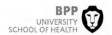

Stage 4. Rebuilding

At this stage the change is embedded and becomes part of the organisation.

These emotional and behavioural reactions apply to you as an individual as much as anyone else. So looking out for them in yourself is important as well.

Recognising what stage individuals and groups of individuals are at can help you tailor your approach and hence reduce stress, for you and for them.

Case study

I thought it was going to be a simple process. I needed to reorganise the office space for the team. We were a total of 40 staff delivering General Practice and communication skills teaching to the medical school. We had had an increase in staff and roles had changed so it was, I thought, only logical to relocate some staff closer to colleagues they would now be working with. I discussed this with the senior admin person and I soon realised that there was going to be a lot of resistance to the moves. People who had shared an office for years were being split up and others who had a single office for years were going to have to work in an open plan office. We sat down and used the change curve to start to plan what we said and to whom. The fact that we predicted certain members of staff would react in an angry manner made it easier for the team I was leading to plan and more importantly cope with the reaction.

One of the key issues when progressing up the hierarchy in any portfolio, and this applies equally to medical education, is that the 'higher' up in the organisation you move the more isolated and lonely you can feel. This is well recognised in any organisation. If you feel you are carrying all of the responsibility for the entire organisation the more isolated you will feel. That is when you perhaps won't want to burden family and friends with the issues but this is when peer support is very useful. This is about looking around for like-minded individuals at the same level as you, individuals who will understand and empathise with the sort of stresses you are facing.

Case study

It struck me on the first week of my new role as Dean of Education in my medical school, where I had worked for ten years, that I was being treated differently by colleagues who I had worked with for a few years. I was now 'the boss' but didn't see myself as that. At the end of the first year in the role I did become increasingly aware that the boss's role was quite lonely. I did feel isolated from the senior team to a certain extent. I tried talking through some of the changes I felt we needed to make to the curriculum but some of my colleagues expressed negativity and there was clearly a vested interest approach going on. That's when I realised I really needed to be discussing these changes and how I might go about them with peers, some at the same level, someone or more than one person grappling with the same sorts of issues. I consciously targeted a number of medical education conferences so as to run into peers and after a few tentative conversations it was clear there were three of us in similar situations and were grappling with similar problems. The three of us have remained a peer support group for the last six years or so and they have helped me cope, not giving me answers, but knowing that there are others struggling with the same issues does help me to cope better and keep going.

Feeling isolated is different to actually being disjoined from the organisation. The latter can lead to you not understanding the impact of decisions and then making decisions that can't be delivered, leading to loss of trust from staff and a spiral of further isolation.

If there is evidence of isolation of you and your team there are recognised strategies that can help reduce that. It has to be recognised that you can never eliminate the isolation but minimise it.

Decentralised decision-making

Different tactics have been described that are argued to reduce the risks of isolation. One such tactic is to essentially decentralise decision-making and therefore accountability at lower levels within the organisation. The argument is that in most organisations, and this will apply to medical education environments, lower levels are able to react in a faster and more agile manner than at higher

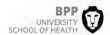

levels. This is clearly in part because they are closer to the real issues which require solutions. Of course you will need to ensure within the organisation you are now responsible for that those levels are staffed with competent and confident individuals.

Of course there is a 'cost' to this, in that this increased efficiency and decision-making will require assessment of competency of staff at those levels and undoubtedly ongoing training requirements.

There are of course risks with decentralisation of budget and decision-making, the first of which is that it can then become more difficult to make decisions in a collaborative and integrated fashion across the different silos as they develop. In addition, decentralisation in its purest form can lead to the exclusion of those at a higher level from having input into issues, solutions and decision-making.

Institute top to bottom interaction

This approach is complementary to decentralisation, in that the top of the organisation encourages, facilitates and rewards decentralisation of decision-making, but also ensures that there is a clear two-way communication between the top and the bottom. It is essential to set up processes to listen across the organisation as well.

The concept of 'managing by walking about' is an example of this tactic in action. One of the purposes of this approach of enhanced top to bottom co-interaction is to lead to a point where there is increased trust by both upper and lower levels of each other's competence and good intentions.

Of course these tactics can only work if there are not too many hierarchical levels within the organisation. So as you move up the medical education career path what you will need to do is look at the number of levels within your vertical hierarchy and if possible (if you can influence this) reduce the number of levels. In diagrammatic terms you need to move from a relatively tall and narrow pyramid to a much shorter and broader structure within the organisation.

BPP
UNIVERSITY
SCHOOL OF HEALTH

Case study

One of the most difficult things I had to face when I first took up the role of Associate Medical Director for Education in my Trust was the issue of so many small decisions that I had to deal with on a day to day basis. These ranged from signing off all trainee doctors' study leave forms to deciding which consultants got what money to support their CPD plans and so on. This was overwhelming. I spent the first three months not actually doing the job but signing bits of paper. When I asked why this was the case I was told: it's the way we have always done it. The implication was very clear … if that's the way we have always done it, that's the way we were going to continue to do it. The issue I had was that all of these decisions, although important, were not what the job was about. The job was enhancing the quality of learning for all doctors in the Trust. I found it increasingly frustrating and did wonder if I had made the right choice. In the end I decided that I needed to devolve authority down to departments and College Tutors and set out principles for them to make those decisions. All I asked for was a biannual report showing how much had been spent and where and what happened as a result. Devolving these day to day decisions down to staff better placed to make them enabled me to have the headroom to focus on the strategic issues facing the Trust.

Horizontal relationships

One of the stresses you may face as you move up the tree is the concept and practical reality of silos in the organisation. In any organisation a silo can be one department, or a geographical group if located from others, if you are on separate sites. Silos form when employees develop loyalty to the group/subgroup rather than the organisation/employer. As silos embed members become more fixed, resistant to change and insular. In addition, members of a silo tend to start to think alike and behave in a similar manner. So if you are trying to innovate, which in a medical education role you will be (or should be), it can be a challenge to innovate silos.

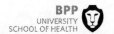

In regard to innovation:

> *It must be remembered that there is nothing more difficult to carry out, or doubtful of success or dangerous to handle, than to initiate a new order of things. For the initiator has the enmity of all those who profit by the old order, and only lukewarm defenders in all those who would benefit by the new order* (Niccolò Machiavelli, 1513)

So collaboration, sharing of ideas and innovation will require you to be aware of any current or growing silos and taking steps to minimise them otherwise your role/job will be more difficult.

Case study

I had been a Senior Lecturer in my medical school for a number of years and then was promoted to be Programme Director with overall responsibility for the four-year graduate entry programme. A part of what was needed was a generic continuing professional development (CPD) programme, teaching the teachers essentially. When I started to discuss this with different teams there was significant resistance. Staff doing the same job had different job titles, General Practitioners, Consultants and non-clinical lecturers. Each unit had different approaches to leave, working from home policies and different levels of budget for CPD and some had a policy on CPD and others didn't. It struck me that these inconsistent practices didn't make sense and were unfair. When I started discussing these with the individual departments they were resistant to any consideration of change. The problem was silos. I had heard of the silos before, but now I saw it in action and it was a barrier to me doing my job. So, with the help of my business manager we devised a plan to initially describe all the different practices on paper and show it to all leads within each of the areas. With this we described a co-ordinated package for supporting all staff in CPD mapped to their educational role and asked each to comment on this. It did become clear to some leads that the plan would be of benefit to them. The key was showing the evidence from elsewhere that having a more standardised approach benefited everyone.

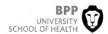

Mentoring

Much has been written about mentoring in medicine. Some Royal Colleges support mentoring schemes and a lot of Health Boards/ Trusts, Medical Schools and Deaneries offer mentoring opportunities. There are many definitions of mentoring but a simple one offered by Megginson and Clutterbuck (1995) is as follows:

> *Help by one person to another in making significant transitions in knowledge, work or thinking*

Broadly speaking there are two types of mentorship relationship, informal and formal. Within the latter it may be that within the organisation you work there may be a scheme whereby individuals are identified as potential mentors and are trained and work to a certain set of rules. Irrespective of the type of relationship, formal or informal, the key element is that the mentee ie you seeking the mentor will drive the agenda. In more formal and systematic approaches there are typically rules of engagement which involve the following:

1. You as the mentee decide on the frequency and type of communication ie face to face, email, telephone.

2. The mentor acts as a sounding board and does not advise or tell you what to do.

3. There is a two-way relationship within any mentor/mentee relationship ie there is mutual respect.

4. The relationship is characterised as 'a relationship between equals' (Hay, 1999). The mentoring relationship can be short term and task focused, therefore similar to executive coaching, but more often than not it refers to a longer-term mentoring relationship rather than a one-off focused relationship.

5. One of the main purposes of the relationship is that you as the mentee are to be helped to maximise your potential both in terms of what you do on a day to day basis and in terms of career aspirations.

There is a bit of a health warning whenever you are seeking a mentor, typically the informal mentors fall out of collaborative and constructive relationships, ie in a clinical setting. You have to be aware that the mentor/mentee relationship can potentially become quite destructive; this has been described by David Clutterbuck (2004) as the 'toxic mentor', characterised by the following:

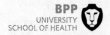

1. The mentor rushes around helping others, rather than addressing their own needs.

2. The mentor brings their issues and problems to the relationship.

3. The mentor has an alternative agenda that does not map to the mentees.

4. The mentor takes profound offence when the mentee does not follow their advice.

5. As above the mentor frequently gives the mentee advice and tells them what to do.

In order to help you survive within your medical education portfolio career it is worthwhile recognising these characteristics when choosing either formal or informal mentor relationships.

Any mentor, formal or informal, should understand frameworks and models to help the mentee and one is the skills helper model. It is useful for you to be aware of this model in that you should be the recipient of this approach and if you recognise it this will give you a level of assurance that the mentor knows what they are doing.

Case study

When I first became a consultant the Trust did offer a mentoring scheme and I really didn't understand what it was about and therefore didn't bother with it. It was only really after about three or four years I was getting more involved in teaching medical students and started to think that I needed to take this role more seriously. I found myself asking more 'senior' colleagues who were in formal medical education leadership roles. These networks formed and in essence have turned into an informal mentor type relation. Now I understand the process (because of studying a Master's in medical education); I use these three informal people more effectively. I do use them as a sounding board, not asking them what I should do. That's my decision. Why these relationships have stood the test of time is that I trust each of them not to break confidentiality. So, I feel I can share my plans and aspirations and talk about difficult, actually stressful things that have happened or plan ahead for things that I know are coming. I see my informal mentors as lifelong professional and also personal support.

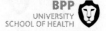

Executive coaching

Executive coaching is mainly associated with one to one relationships. It is argued effective coaching supports personal changes and growth and therefore your personal effectiveness. Coaching is about helping the individual to get the best out of themselves and therefore has a similar generic aim to mentoring. With mentoring as described above, the focus is on the broader individual, more likely than not over a longer period of time. It is argued that there are two central aims of coaching. The first is awareness, which is described above and the second is accountability. By this we mean that the executive coaching will enable you to accept and recognise greater levels of personal responsibility for your communication, engagement and interaction with people and environments around you. This will improve your understanding of the environment you are working in as well as those people around you increasing their understanding of your role.

In essence, executive coaching tends to be a task- or problem-focused approach and as such if you are faced with a particular issue/problem that is a trigger to explore executive coaching.

There are many models that are used to structure task-/goal-orientated conversations; one such is the GROW model (Whitmore, 1999). It is a model used by professional coaches but you can use the steps yourself.

Goal: what is your goal? How committed are you to this?

Reality: what is the current reality? Where am I now?

Options and obstacles: what are my options and what is stopping or delaying me getting to where I want to be?

Will: what is the plan? What do I need to do to achieve my goal?

There are certain rules to starting with an executive coach, the first of which is to be clear about the specific problem/challenge you have and the potential solutions. It is important to create a contract; that is, you are clear about what you want to get out of the sessions and the coach is clear about what they are able to provide. Part of what you will need to do is to explore alternative options/solutions and the accepting of the need to possibly look outside the current solutions that you are currently considering. It is important that any executive coaching session belongs to you.

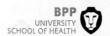

There are many forms of executive coaching and much confusion with mentoring. Informal relationship is perhaps closer to mentoring but formal executive coaching can be very positive at helping maintain your resilience.

It is best to see the use of a coach as helping you achieve a specific personal or professional goal and so it is time limited and task orientated.

Case study

I was finding it difficult to move from a Deputy Dean of Medical Education in my local medical school to becoming the Dean. I had applied for the role previously but hadn't been appointed. Advice from some friends outside of medicine was that I would be best to apply for a Dean's role in another medical school elsewhere in the country. Through my appraisals it was suggested that executive coaching may help. It did.

The opportunity to talk though and reflect on my current position, where I wanted to be and what I needed to do to get there helped me see that I needed a number of things, one of which was a higher UK profile in a specific area. I had up to that point developed my medical education career around or based on the principle that I knew a little, or a moderate amount about most things. A jack of all trades. I always had a specific interest in professionalism in general and as a result of the coaching I then focused some time on developing this area in my own school but also disseminating the work through conferences. It is impossible to say that the coaching did the trick but it did help.

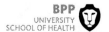

Chapter summary

There are a range of tools and approaches you can use to survive in a medical education career. These are generic approaches and apply to all, although some will suit you as an individual better than others. The more tools in your toolbox the better.

Key points

- Individual skills to improve your resilience are important.
- Develop your ability to reflect on your decisions.
- You will manage and lead change.
- Improve your decision-making.
- Watch out for silos in your organisation.
- Seek out informal or formal mentors.
- Explore executive coaching.

Useful resources

Bandura, A (1997) *Self-efficacy: The Exercise of Control.* New York: W. H. Freeman & Co Ltd.

Carkhuff, RR (2000) *The Art of Helping in the 21st Century.* Amherst, MA: Human Resource Development Press.

Egan, G (2007) *The Skilled Helper.* 8th edition. Boston, MA: Brooks Cole.

Morton-Cooper, A and Palmer, A (1993) *Mentoring in Action.* London: Kogan Page.

References

Carver, CS. Resilience and thriving: Issues, models, and linkages. *Journal of Social Issues* 1998; 54(2): 245–266.

Clutterbuck, D (2004) *Everyone needs a mentor.* UK: CIPD.

Goleman, D. Leadership that gets results. *Harvard Business Review* 2000; Mar–Apr: 78–90.

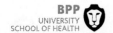
BPP
UNIVERSITY
SCHOOL OF HEALTH

Hay, J (1999) *Transformational Mentoring – Creating Developmental Alliances for Changing Organizational Cultures*. Watford: Sherwood Publishing.

Kluber-Ross, E (1997) *On Death and Dying*. New York: Scribner Publishing Group.

Megginson, D and Clutterbuck, D (1995) *Mentoring in Action*. London: Kogan Page.

Whitmore, J (2009) *Coaching for performance*. 4th edition. London: Nicholas Brealey.

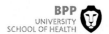

Chapter 9

The future of medical education in the workplace

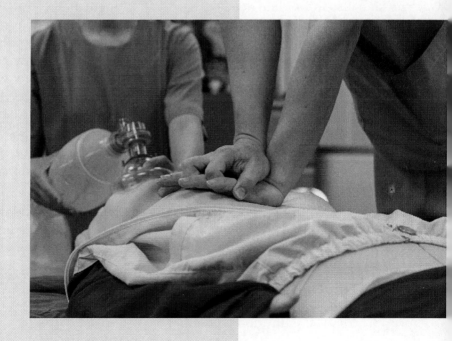

Introduction

Medical education has taken great strides over the last few years but still has a long way to go to get the full recognition of its real contribution to patient care and safety. The introduction of professional standards for both undergraduate and postgraduate educators has gone a long way to establish and professionalise the role within all Local Education Providers (LEPs). The need for appropriate appointments systems, continuing professional development (CPD) and appraisals have again altered the perception of the role of the educator. There is wide recognition of the published work that shows that organisations that have the best training also have the best patient outcomes. There are a number of key questions to be asked by each LEP, including:

- Is an education lead represented at board level?
- What is the status of education and reporting to the board of an LEP?
- What actual investment does the organisation make in educational provision?

Clearly some of these issues have not moved on despite the evidence of the benefits of educational engagement, not only for patient care but also individual development, recruitment and retention of the entire workforce. There is, however, a wider interest in medical education and its processes that will shape the future direction and raise the profile of the subject. The financial investment alone would be enough to ensure this but it is also about new ways of working and providing a sustainable workforce for the NHS.

What are the issues that will therefore shape the future strategic direction of medical education? These will clearly be across the undergraduate/postgraduate divide but will be much further reaching with a much greater focus on the multiprofessional team and new ways of working.

The following gives an outline of current thinking and developments that are in train and will deliver into the workforce going forward. They also have major implications for the specialty of medical education. The areas we will discuss are:

1. Generalist training
2. Medical Licensing Assessment
3. Medical education credential

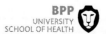

4. Education contracts for trainees
5. Revalidation and relicensing
6. New medical schools
7. Education membership organisations
8. Multiprofessional education
9. Technology and education
10. Finance

1. Generalist training

When considering the future of medical education it is perhaps pertinent to start with the 'Shape of Training' report (Greenaway, 2013), a comprehensive review of postgraduate training. The report was published in October 2013 and consisted of 19 recommendations. The major focus was on whether training should be more generalist than specialist and therefore whether it could be shortened and more flexible. The generalist debate focuses on the ability of the doctor to take a more holistic view of the patient rather than perhaps the reductionist specialty or sub-specialty approach. A more generalist training approach would allow more doctors to have the skills work on the 'front door' of the hospital which has come under increasing pressure over the years. That we would clearly still need to have specialists and super-specialists is not questioned but exactly how many are needed and where they should be working certainly is. The move to having larger tertiary centres covering a larger geographical patch and focusing the resources is certainly the way forward. The training implications in adopting this service delivery approach are far reaching. While the majority of doctors would undertake the majority of their training in District General Hospitals there would have to be specific centres capable of delivering sub-specialty training reflecting the workforce needs of the NHS.

The report has already been discussed in Chapter 7; however, it is worth noting that none of the Royal Colleges felt that their training programmes could be shortened and indeed General Practice has been lobbying for a longer period of training for some years. The role of credentials for sub-specialty training was viewed with some anxiety, with the expressed concern that this approach would create a sub-consultant role. There remain unanswered questions such as who would fund any credentials and whether there is a risk that we would just have a plethora of credentials and 'badge collectors'.

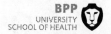

The Royal College of Surgeons has proposed a series of pilots with the aim of improving general surgery skills, in line with the 'shape model'. There is currently uncertainty as to the timing, detail and funding of these pilots.

2. Medical Licensing Assessment

This was one of the 'Shape of Training' recommendations – that there should be a defined standard and common finals examination for medical students across the UK. At present the GMC reviews curricula and assessments that each separate medical school has in place and accredits them individually. While they have to adhere to what is required in the standards the methods used by each medical school in the UK can be very different. The GMC now feels that this lack of standardisation does not give the public confidence that all those that pass finals are of a similar standard across the UK. The introduction of a Medical Licensing Assessment (MLA) would potentially help towards a resolution. The other major issue with the MLA is that it could set the standard for those non-UK doctors who wish to work in this country by ensuring they sat this assessment prior to taking up employment. As it currently stands the UK is unable to test any European Union doctors who have obtained a primary medical qualification in their own country. The UK has to recognise their qualification and is unable to test their language skills. This is a patient safety issue and may of course be resolved post-Brexit. In the future, it might be politically and financially difficult to invest in a new MLA that only the UK and non-EU doctors would have to sit. It will take a great deal of work and expense to realise this vision, which does not solve the issue that we need to ensure the standards of all doctors from any country have the requisite knowledge and skills to work in the NHS.

Medical schools in the UK for some time have used a common bank of questions as part of their final examinations. These have been a small, but growing, proportion of the examinations. Preliminary results do show that there is a great disparity in the marks across the medical schools (Taylor et al, 2017) which perhaps does reinforce the need for a uniform UK assessment process. The GMC has formally consulted on the MLA and we await further developments.

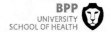

3. Medical education credential

When is a specialty not a specialty? What part of the working week do you get paid for doing a professional job but have no defined standards, curricula or transparent career progression? The answer is clearly when you are involved in medical education. New standards have come into place via the GMC but individuals get programmed activities for undertaking education the same as they get paid for their direct clinical work. Medical education is not considered a specialty, indeed it cannot even be considered a sub-specialty since it has no host specialty. This does pose a dilemma for the continued professionalisation of this important aspect of the working week.

The Academy of Medical Educators (AoME) has been developing a credential in medical education and this may be the way forward to obtain proper recognition with a registrable qualification on the medical register. The purpose of the medical education credential would be to attract all those that have a number of contracted sessions in their job plan in education to work towards a defined standard of practice and demonstrate that they achieve this standard in the workplace. It is very much about demonstrating the educational skills in the workplace and is not just restricted to doctors but anyone who is involved in delivering teaching and training to medical students or doctors. While the GMC has already agreed on the need for credentials in clinical specialties, it would have to agree on the need to have a qualification added to the medical register. This would be a voluntary exercise for individuals but the ultimate hope is that it would be seen as a 'must have' qualification for all those perusing a portfolio career in medical education.

Pilots are already underway to hone the work that would need to be done to demonstrate the skills required to obtain the credential. An individual would have to demonstrate that they had acquired the knowledge commensurate with the subject. This could be attendance at an accredited course or possession of a higher qualification in medical education.

The real bulk of the work for the medical education credential is demonstrating how that knowledge is delivered by keeping a portfolio of evidence and submitting this for assessment. The portfolio looks to cover the domains described in the AoME standards in Chapter 6 (see Table 9.1).

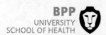

Academy of Medical Educators (AoME) practice domains
1. Designing and planning learning
2. Teaching and facilitating learning
3. Assessment of learning
4. Educational research and scholarship
5. Educational management and leadership

Table 9.1 Academy of Medical Educators (AoME) practice domains

It is envisaged that to meet the requirements of the medical education credential you will have to provide evidence of your actions within each domain and, as you do in appraisal now, reflect on those activities. This develops your portfolio of 'evidence of action'. This portfolio will be underpinned by a knowledge base (Table 9.2) where you again provide evidence of your knowledge being put into action at a practical (practice) level or at a policy level.

Those seeking a medical education credential should know about:
The role of statutory or regulatory bodies in medical education
How educational leadership relates to professional practice as an educator
Models of curriculum design
Methods of learning
Methods of teaching
Giving feedback
How to engage learners in active participation

Table 9.2 Examples of knowledge base potentially required for medical education credential

Figure 9.1 (with permission from AoME) is from a draft version of the portfolio and gives you a sense of what might be expected within the domain of Educational Research and Scholarship.

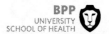

Educational Research and Scholarship

Standard Level 2	Please provide evidence of your application of the theoritical and evidence-base of medical education. For example, educational activity to which you have applied medical education theory or evidence might relate to clinician educator role in primary or secondary care, clinical skills tutoring, communication skills teaching etc. Log your application of educational research and scholarship using the grid below. We would normally expect these to be at level 2 within a variety of roles and settings.
4.2.1 4.2.1 understands and applies a range of educational theories and principles **4.2.2** Critically evaluates the educational literature and applies this learning to his or her educational practice **4.2.3** Participates in the design and deelopment of educational programmes, projects or research **4.2.4** Interprets and applies the results of educational research to his or her educational practice	

Figure 9.1 Academy of Medical Educators proposed medical education credential – requirements under the domain of Educational Research and Scholarship

The reflective element to the portfolio is clearly very important and is in line with the principles of revalidation. Much of this evidence can also therefore be used in that process by just cutting and pasting. Many established educators will already have the evidence required to fulfil the criteria as outlined in the portfolio but those coming new to the subject could expect to gather the evidence over a period of between one and two years.

The standards and development of the portfolio may not be suitable for those that only undertake educational supervision but for all those with more substantial portfolios in education it can be seen as a clear marker of the professional work that they undertake.

The standards are similar to those that the AoME uses for its entry requirements for membership and fellowship. These again are the backbone of the standards for educators that the GMC has established for its educator quality framework. This alignment prevents duplication of work and establishes a clear understanding of what this 'specialty' is seeking to achieve. Time will tell if this is the established way of ensuring standards across the UK and if this approach obtains traction with medical educators.

Another important point is that as these standards are generic they could form the basis of a multiprofessional approach to education within the NHS. Adoption by other professions would again ensure consistency across the educational environment. The fact that only doctors would get the credential on their entry in the medical register is a small issue and perhaps of little interest to other health workers but the unification of standards and approach will benefit everyone involved in education.

4. Education contracts for trainees

Every doctor in training currently is asked to sign an employment contract when they start a new job with either the hospital or GP practice. This should cover the contractual service elements of the job eg pay, hours to be worked, holiday entitlement. However, trainees do not currently have an education contract that outlines what they can expect to receive and contribute to for their own education. A new initiative from the Wales Deanery is the implementation of education contracts for all specialties. The Education Contract is a formal agreement between the Trainee, Wales Deanery, Welsh Government and the relevant Health Board or Trust. The agreed criteria and metrics for the Education Contract are mapped against GMC-approved specialty curricula and Standards for Medical Education and Training which came into effect in January 2016. The contract stipulates a commitment from the Health Boards and Trusts to ensure trainees have access to the required number of outpatient clinics, theatre sessions, teaching sessions, ward rounds and other educational opportunities to meet training needs. The specific requirements of each trainee are monitored via a web-based app tool where the trainee can log attendance at key learning opportunities. This education contract attendance system is a live monitoring tool that allows early warning of any issues that could compromise the quality of training and that are then escalated to the LEP immediately and can be resolved quickly. There is a real opportunity for this approach to be rolled out to the rest of the UK as an example of the importance of the investment in training that the Deaneries/Local Education and Training Boards (LETBs) on behalf of the health departments need to ensure is maximised.

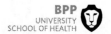

5. Revalidation and relicensing

The current process of revalidation and relicensing has already been covered in Chapter 7. However, the long lead-in period to ensure that everyone has gone through at least one cycle does not finish until 2018. The GMC is committed to reviewing the process and evaluating what has been achieved by this new initiative. What may we expect as a result of the evaluation? What changes might we expect going forward? Clearly this will be about evolution rather than revolution as while the yearly cycle of appraisals contributes to the evidence the individual will only have relicensed once so far. The positive aspects of the process are:

- The engagement of the individual
- Yearly mandatory appraisal process
- 360 degree feedback on performance
- The reflective nature of the portfolio
- Up to date CPD programmes
- Forward planning of aims and objectives for the next year
- Coverage of all roles in the job plan

These are some of the aspects that would be hard to say should not always have been in place. Perhaps the negative aspect of the process is the additional paperwork and time to complete the process, not helped by computer glitches along the way. There is a more fundamental question that will come out in the review and that is whether it is doing what it was supposed to do, namely giving patients confidence in the ability of their doctor and identifying those who are underperforming. At a macro level we will know how many doctors have been denied relicensing and the reasons for this. We will also know how many have been deferred and again the reasons for this. If the process is going to continue (and it will) there may be more to gain from looking at the areas that are causing doctors to fail the process rather than the majority who will relicense without any issues. This would have training and educational implications and may help make the entire process more streamlined and focused on the standards required of all doctors.

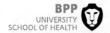

6. New medical schools

There are several new medical schools springing up across the UK which are essentially private. They are not there because of any government request to produce more schools; however, NHS England has announced a 1,500 increase in medical student numbers. There are several reasons for this current situation. The private medical schools are responding to a perceived need that many students with appropriate grades fail to currently get into an established medical school, that overseas students are keen to study medicine in this country, that there are sufficient people willing to pay the fees and that it may enhance the reputation of the affiliated university to have an undergraduate medical department. NHS England, on the other hand, has increased training numbers in response to the need to make the NHS less reliant on overseas doctors to deliver its service in the NHS. At present almost 1,500 doctors who finish the UK Foundation Programme do not immediately go into core training. This is a significant gap, which translates currently to poor uptake of posts in general medicine, emergency medicine, paediatrics, General Practice and psychiatry. This will result in a reduced Consultant and GP workforce further down the line.

While the increase in medical student numbers is to be welcomed, whether from the private schools or otherwise, it leaves a more fundamental question about the role of the medical schools in the delivery of the future workforce for the NHS and the large investment needed to train medical students to qualification.

There are those who believe that the role of medical schools is not to produce doctors for the NHS but to produce clinician scientists. There is no doubt that clinician scientists are needed to drive forward the research agenda and certainly a percentage of doctors need to fulfil that role. However, the percentage is small compared to that needed for front line patient care. The changing demographics mean we need to train doctors for an elderly population with multiple co-morbidities, polypharmacy and degrees of cognitive impairment. They need to understand the fiscal restraints of the system and find new ways of working and delivering a patient-focused service. How far the medical schools have a regard for this and reflect that in their curricula is a challenge. The move to an MLA may allow greater input into what the service and patients actually need in

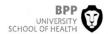

a modern NHS and therefore assessment would drive learning to areas that are responsive to need. The introduction of private medical schools may well influence the proportion of teaching in the community and lean towards producing more doctors who are skilled and want to work outside the secondary care system. Will we see medical schools only producing community physicians or clinical academics? If an organisation does not get the workers with the skills it requires to function then it might decide to train them itself or specifically commission focused training for their needs. This will change the way medical schools react to the educational enviroment and force a greater collaboration between themselves and the employers. Indeed, it would be fair to say that when asked the employers invariably say they want more of the same. Real strategic vision and an overview are difficult for employers to achieve when the main priority is always balancing the books in any one financial year. Long-term investment, particularly in staff and new ways of working, are slow to be introduced. This has left training organisations to continue producing the same product with little inclination to engage in the debate about new kinds of doctors and training. The future will need a much more inclusive transparent debate on where we need to be and how that might be achieved. The lead-in times in training run past a decade so planning change has to be bold with a commitment from all parties.

7. Education membership organisations

There are many organisations that have been set up to represent the interests of certain groups of medical educators and some include:

- AoME, which has set the standards for medical education embraced by the GMC

- Association for the Study of Medical Education, which leans towards medical education researchers

- National Association of Clinical Tutors, which delivers educational provision for tutors in the workplace

- Association for Simulated Practice in Healthcare, which encompasses medical education using simulation in all its forms

To the above one could add the Higher Education Academy, Centre for the Advancement of Interprofessional Education, other

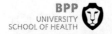

health professional education bodies and indeed the education departments of all the Royal Colleges. Does this plethora of bodies actually advance the specialty of medical education? Are they representative of those involved in the day to day delivery of education or are they just niche organisations that deliver a part of the educational agenda?

Membership of any of these organisations is voluntary and requires an annual fee, so the individual is making a positive choice to be a member. Each organisation hosts annual conferences and CPD events and have regular electronic communication with their members. There is, however, little cross-communication between the organisations. They all compete with each other for members, keynote conference speakers, research grants and influence at a national level. While some of the above are multiprofessional, doctors are still the dominant members. The organisations mainly survive on the membership fees and have little real infrastructure, being reliant on the goodwill of those that serve on their councils and give up their time.

If medical education is to be fully recognised for the specialty it is and the contribution it makes to patient care then the diversity of all these organisations does not help achieve that aim going forward. Medical education needs to be at the centre of any debate on new ways of working, changing roles in the NHS, workforce planning and multiprofessional delivery of healthcare. But to whom would a health department go to get such advice and be reassured that they had spoken to a representative, an authoritative body? Surely, the time has come for a new model of representation for medical education, one that has an overarching structure encompassing the individual niche organisations but representing them all. It could be recognised as the place to go to get expert advice, to respond to government consultations, to draw in all those involved in medical education making them part of a bigger picture organisation. This would stop the competition for membership, speakers and research grants and allow the central body to work on behalf of all and truly have a seat at the top tables to input into the future education and structure of the NHS.

The Developing Excellence in Medical Education conference was a starting point in bringing together all those organisations that are delivering medical education. It is held every two years and has successfully brought the education population together for this two-day conference that shares innovation and best practice. Further collaborative work would be a good starting point but bringing everyone together under one umbrella must be the ultimate aim. There are examples of this type of federation model that allows individual organisations to continue delivering their areas of expertise, namely in Canada (Association of Faculties of Medicine of Canada), and indeed the Academy of Royal Colleges in the UK uses a similar approach to represent all colleges at a national level.

Medical educationalists need to be ambitious and push for education to sit side by side with all other specialties and have the representative voice required to improve its status in the workplace, within the LEPs and nationally to acquire the funding needed to deliver the highest quality of teaching and training that patients would benefit from.

8. Multiprofessional education

While the focus of this book has been on how to be a medical educator and hence principally about doctors in educational roles, it is important to acknowledge that the future is about a multiprofessional approach to all aspects of education and service delivery. Much has been spoken and written about a more integrated approach to all aspects of healthcare for many decades but we are still far short of delivering a truly integrated approach. If medical education had an overarching federation then there could be a unification of the standards of educational delivery across all professions. The educational environment would become a reality and common skills training for all educationalists would be the norm. Professions could then sit side by side for many generic elements of their own curricula and skills training. There are currently 11 health and social care regulators across the UK. Each profession must be a member of its professional regulation body. Each of these regulators has its own professional standards, which must be adhered to by its members. Central government has already announced that these regulatory bodies should merge in some form to get a more consistent approach to professional standards. This is certainly true for medical education and a great step forward would be the agreement and amalgamation of the current educational standards across the professions. This is probably the step that would finally push a truly meaningful multiprofessional educational delivery.

9. Technology and education

The future will clearly see advances in technology that will have to be incorporated into the curricula. Better simulation packages, smartphone technology, bedside knowledge assistance are all already in use in some shape or form across the UK. The future is much more about knowledge management than any idea that one person can know all about their own specialty. While there will always be a place for face to face teaching and patient-focused teaching, distance learning and using only the best lecturers and demonstrators bring teaching onto a global scale. The ability to learn from watching the best performers globally, the real sharing of best practice and of critical incidents from those leading the field before the procedures are taken up locally can only be a benefit to patient care. Health is a global subject and so is medical education but too much of it is duplicated rather than time spent advancing the subject in an evidence-based way.

10. Finance

It would be remiss not to mention finances and medical education, particularly in these days of continued financial austerity. Medical education funding will have to take its share of any efficiency savings, the same as services. This does focus the mind on new ways of working and reviewing the working patterns and employment of those in medical education. Many organisational structures have been in place for decades and reviewing how effective they continue to be is an exercise well worth doing if only to confirm that the best and financially efficient processes are in place. The investment in education is multimillions of pounds, most of which supports the training grade salaries. The formula for paying these was historically at the mid-point of the scale but that is clearly not a true reflection of the costs. The out of hours payments are also the responsibility of the employer rather than the Deanery and again shows marked variation depending on rota commitments.

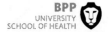

The remaining educational budget is largely on staffing costs at the Deanery and infrastructure costs at postgraduate centres, library costs and various CPD events.

There are two aspects of the budget that need a global review.

1. Is the LEP giving value for money for the training budget they receive?

2. Are the internal Deanery/LETB processes efficient and value for money?

The commissioning visits should inform the medical schools and the Postgraduate Deanery if the LEP is committed to training and offering the requisite educational environment. In the postgraduate arena the Deanery also needs to engage with the LEPs in understanding the true cost of training, including locum cover, banding payments and cost of any new contract (currently in England). This is not necessarily to bid for new monies but to get an accurate picture of the costings to reflect back to the relevant Departments of Health.

With regard to the Postgraduate Deanery infrastructure perhaps the first place to review is the hierarchical tiers in the education structure, many of which will be historic. Does the Deanery want dozens of educators on a small number of sessions or are there economies of scale that could be achieved by amalgamating sessions so fewer individuals have more sessions? This would also help professionalise the educator role and enable the Deanery to offer more support in the development of those individuals. In GP vocational training do you need a GP trainer, a Course Organiser, a Regional Organiser and a Head of GP School? Is there scope for less individuals on more sessions and therefore greater efficiency?

What should a Deanery team look like going forward? Clearly the argument should be that the medical education infrastructure should be leaner with a core workforce and a more substantial number of sessions emphasising the professional nature of the role.

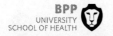

Chapter summary

The future of medical education is bright. It has moved forward greatly in the last few years thanks to directives on educational standards by the GMC, the introduction of revalidation and relicensing, the introduction of generic professional capabilities and the greater flexibility of the approach to teaching and training. More work is required to integrate the other health professions into common standards and ensure a common educational environment for all. Better use of technologies and only showing the best examples of how to undertake procedures or expert teachers and lecturers will also come to the fore.

The MLA, new ways of delivering the undergraduate curriculum and greater input from the employers will all ensure a better, safer, more patient-focused NHS for the future.

Key points

- Medical education needs to continue to professionalise its role.
- Educational standards should apply across all health professions.
- Financial constraints should act as a trigger for new ways of working.
- Technology and best practice is still under-utilised and disseminated.
- Trainees need transparent, deliverable education contracts.

Useful resources

Academy of Medical Educators – www.medicaleducators.org

Association of Faculties of Medicine of Canada – https://afmc.ca/

Wales Deanery – www.walesdeanery.org

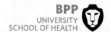

References

Gurnell M, Johnson, N, Kluth D et al. Variation in passing standards for graduation-level knowledge items at UK medical schools. *Medical Education* 2017; 51(6): 612–620.

Greenaway, D (2013) *Shape of Training: Securing the Future of Excellent Patient Care – the Final Report of the Independent Review.* [Online]. Available at: www.shapeoftraining.co.uk/static/documents/content/ Shape_of_training_FINAL_Report.pdf_53977887.pdf [Accessed 21 June 2017].

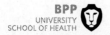

Chapter 9

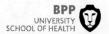

Glossary

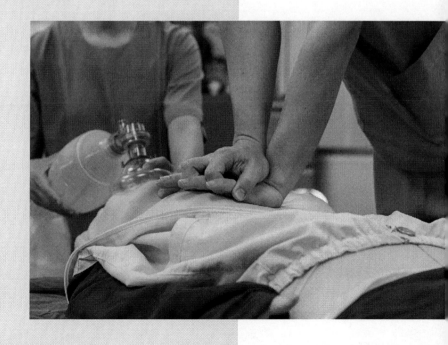

Glossary

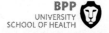

A&E	Accident and Emergency
AMD (Ed)	Associate Medical Director (Education)
AMEE	Association for Medical Education in Europe
AoME	Academy of Medical Educators
ASME	Association for the Study of Medical Education
ASPiH	Association for Simulation Practice in Healthcare
CCT	Certificate of Completion of Training
CEO	Chief Executive Officer
CMO	Chief Medical Officer
CPD	Continuing Professional Development
CT	College Tutor
CV	Curriculum Vitae
DCMO	Deputy Chief Medical Officer
DME	Director of Medical Education
DoMe	Dean of Medical Education
ED	Emergency Department
EM	Emergency Medicine
ENT	Ear Nose and Throat
ES	Educational Supervisor
GMC	General Medical Council
GPC	Generic Professional Capabilities
HEA	Higher Education Academy
HoMS	Head of Medical School
HoSS	Head of Specialty School
LEP	Local Education Provider

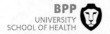

Glossary

LETB	Local Education and Training Board
MBTI	Myers-Briggs Type Indicator
MDT	Multi-disciplinary Team
MSC	Medical Schools Council
NACT	National Association of Clinical Tutors
NSS	National Student Survey
PA	Physicians Assistant
REF	Research Excellence Framework
SMA	Senior Medical Adviser
SMO	Senior Medical Officer
TPD	Training Programme Director
UCAS	Universities and College Admissions Service

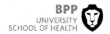

Index

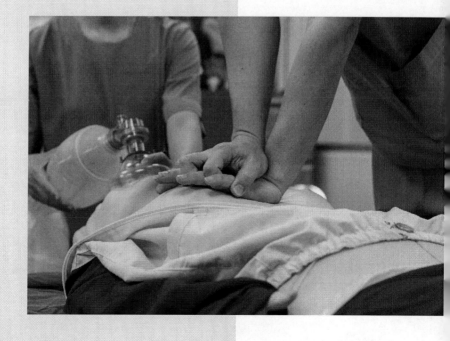

Index

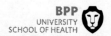

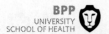

Index

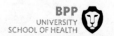

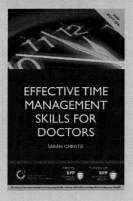
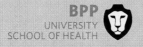

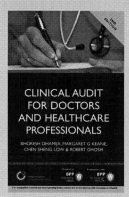
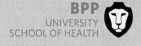

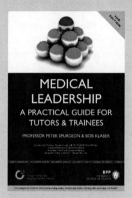
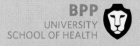

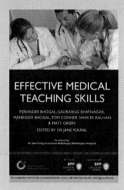
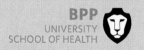

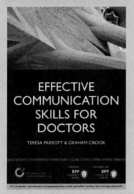
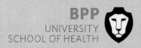

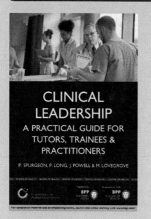
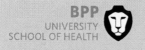